Personal Training

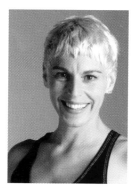

Jennifer Wade
Personal Training

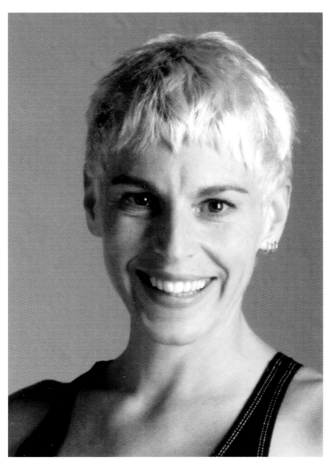

Individual Fitness Programs
& Training Plans for Every Body Type

Sterling Publishing Company, Inc.
New York

*In memory of my parents,
who gave me the courage, strength
and integrity to go after my dreams*

Text by Ute Haas
Edited by Claire Bazinet

Library of Congress Cataloging-in-Publication Data

Wade, Jennifer, [date]
    Personal training : individual fitness programs & training plans for every body type / Jennifer Wade.
        p.   cm.
    Includes index.
    ISBN 0-8069-4201-0
    1. Physical fitness. 2. Exercise. I. Title
    GV481.W12   1998
    613.7—dc21   98–15953
                                                 CIP

10 9 8 7 6 5 4 3 2 1

Published by Sterling Publishing Company, Inc.
387 Park Avenue South, New York, N.Y. 10016
Originally published in Germany and © 1996 by Sudwest Verlag GmbH & Co., Munich
English translation © 1998 by Sterling Publishing Company
Distributed in Canada by Sterling Publishing
c/o Canadian Manda Group, One Atlantic Avenue, Suite 105
Toronto, Ontario, Canada M6K 3E7
Distributed in Great Britain and Europe by Cassell PLC
Wellington House, 125 Strand, London WC2R 0BB, England
Distributed in Australia by Capricorn Link (Australia) Pty Ltd.
P.O. Box 6651, Baulkham Hills, Business Centre, NSW 2153, Australia

Printed in Hong Kong
All rights reserved

Sterling ISBN 0-8069-4201-0

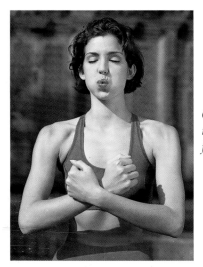

Good breathing technique is essential for strenuous exercise.

Contents

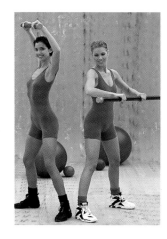

Correct posture and accurate execution are vital for each exercise.

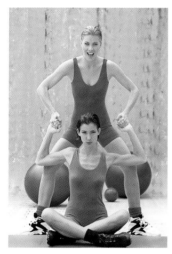

Keep yourself motivated; with a partner or the right music, it's a cinch.

Good luck with your training and have fun with this book!

Jennifer Wade
"My Philosophy"

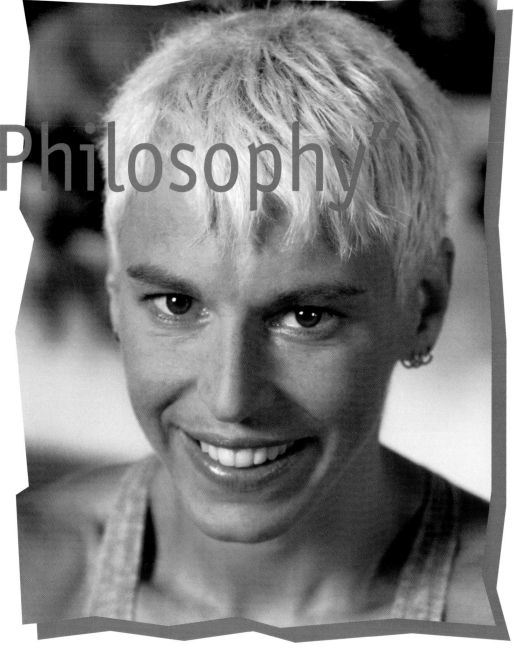

"With my whole heart and the power within me" —that is how I approach fitness. Gemini, the sign of the twins, is not only my Sun sign, but somehow signifies my life. One could say that I have two hearts beating in my soul, one American and one German. Until I was 20 years old I lived in the USA, and I have now lived 23 years in Germany—a simple way of telling you how old I am!

Having grown up in the United States, I experienced and lived through many changes in my country firsthand. Much of what I saw happening about me then, I am reliving now in Germany, giving me a feeling of "deja vu." The fitness trends especially that I grew up with in the USA, I visualized in the German market. So, many of the experiences that I had in my life, I have been able to work through and use to help my clients and guide my students. It has always been important to me to use everything that happens in life: good, bad, positive, and negative as lessons in growth. I believe very strongly that we all have strengths within us...they just must be brought out and used effectively in order to reach the goals we need.

My years of classical ballet taught me incredible discipline and impeccable technique. This, too, I pass on to my clients, my students, and now to you, my readers. I never demand anything from anyone that I would not do myself. All the exercises and programs that I conceived for this book are those that I do myself, teach in my group fitness classes, and give to my personal training clients. My motto is: "I live what I give!"

Whether you believe it or not, I, too, was once at the point in life where now you find yourself. So, with this book I want to become your guide, your own personal trainer. Imagine me standing there beside you, taking your hand, and we will embark on the road to fitness—to finding and developing your inner strength.

Then and Now

When I was growing up in the States, I remember walking to the corner store three or four times a day. My mom walked to the supermarket. If we wanted to mail a letter, we walked to the post office. Now not only do we drive everywhere, we swivel in our chairs to send a fax or send e-mail instead of *going* to the post office. Some people would love simply to drive their car right up to their desk! How many of you out there take the elevator instead of the stairs, or the escalator and *don't* walk up? I mean, when you don't have packages to carry? Be honest now! Most of us leave our movements to technology. Recently home on a visit, I was sad to see how many people live in housing without sidewalks. So even if you *did* want to walk, you couldn't!

Sitting for hours at home in front of the TV set is a major reason why the Surgeon General named a "sedentary lifestyle" as one of the primary contributing factors to heart disease in the United States. And now so many of you have computers to sit in front of! Your "poor" European neighbors, on the other hand, still walk and ride bikes everywhere—into very old age! It's sad to think that one of the richest nations in the world, has the highest rate of cardiovascular disease anywhere!

On top of what this inactivity does to our heart, this "just sitting around" causes a lot of bodily tension—believe it or not! This leads to stiffness and muscular imbalance. Doing the same physical action over and over again, like moving a computer mouse around, also causes imbalances, the so-called overuse syndrome.

"Ah, but I play squash three times a week," you say. Well, here too you are using the same muscles over and over again while other muscles remain relatively under used. Your whole body is not being pushed to its potential. Playing a sport or two is not the same as fitness!

Communication and the media play major roles in our having become so sedentary. With home-order TV, we don't even get up and out to see recent major films.

Instead, our lives are determined by our time planners and calendars. For most of us, daily living is filled with mega-stress. This stress not only makes us nervous, robs us of sleep, keeps us on Prozac, and saps our energy system, but plays havoc with our immune system as well.

The Contradiction—We Know More

The funny thing is that we know more about our bodies and about health than we have ever known. There is such an abundance of health and fitness magazines on the market, television programs with fitness exercises, that we all should be specimens of good health.

If I ask what the bodily problem area is for most people, would you know? I'll bet that, if you are a woman, you'd say the buttocks, thighs or stomach, in that order; the stomach, if you are a man. Well, you might have reason to believe that, but actually the back is the biggest problem area worldwide! Despite all the research and advice out there for correct training and nutrition, most of us have never taken the time or interest to really understand our bodies and its function.

I find it funny that most men, for example, know all about the inner workings of their cars, from the fan belt to the carburetor, but can't even point to it if we ask them to locate their quadriceps muscle. And what about us women? We know which makeup is the best for our skin, but we don't know about the "makeup *under* our skin"— our muscles!

Our body is our home. Just as we know each room and corner of our house, so we should know our organs, muscles, and their functions. As we take care of our homes, we should take care of ourselves—inside as well as outside!

Reach Out!

The fact is: There is no one fast formula to reaching optimal fitness. Changes and improvements should occur in stages, so that they will become a way of life. The most important thing is the decision that you make to take the first step toward a healthy lifestyle. This first step is one you must make alone. The wish to change must come from within you.

In this book, I offer you all my years of experience guiding people, combined with the most up-to-date health and sport science research. Here are tips and ideas from both the American and European point of view; the best of both worlds. A new feeling for life and a positive feeling about yourself are yours for the reading and the doing.

Let me motivate you. Let me "touch your life!"

I. What Does *Fitness* Really Mean?

"I believe in fitness." This short statement is almost always the first thing I say to clients and interviewers. I don't say it just because it sounds good, I say it because I truly believe in the properties of fitness and what it can do for you—because of what it did for me. When I started to write this book, I had to analyze what I really mean when I say those words and why I am so convinced that fitness and being fit can change your life.

If you look in the dictionary, you will find several definitions of "fit." One of them is: "having the right qualifications," another is "worthy or deserving," and another, as we know, is "being in good health." Used in the phrase "having a fit," the word is defined as "an impulsive period of activity or lack of activity." If I go by the dictionary, I could say that if I am fit, I have the right qualifications, am worthy and healthy, and am vacillating between periods of activity and non-activity!

The word "fitness," however, is relatively new to our vocabulary. Yet, even without looking in the dictionary, almost all of us think that being fit means being healthy and strong. But is being healthy only *not* being sick and strong only being able to lift heavy objects?

Fitness encompasses far more than that. Being healthy means having a strong, well-functioning heart, lungs that can take in lots of oxygen, muscles that are well toned and capable of taking on tasks without tiring easily, a body that can bend and stretch without saying "ouch," and a mind that can switch stress off at will. Sounds like an unreachable ideal, doesn't it? Yet each one of us is capable of achieving such goals, or at least improving these areas of our bodies. Becoming fit will not only bring you closer to this state, it will fill you with energy and a strength of will and character that can change your life.

What Is Aerobics?

The word brings to mind Jane Fonda in a leotard, doesn't it? But, in order to prevent cardiovascular disease, strengthen our metabolism and make it more resilient, we should be performing "aerobic" activities such as walking (*not* driving the car), riding a bike (*not* driving the car), and of course, jogging and running.

Aerobics started out as jazz gymnastics, a cute mixture of watered-down jazz movements and calisthenics performed to the top 40 hits of the week. It became a cult with fanatic followers, starting a whole new industry. Aerobics today has become more of

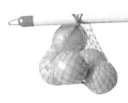

Being Fit—A Lifetime Philosophy

Being fit has to do with body, mind and soul. It means being able to accomplish everyday tasks with ease, not being stressed at the

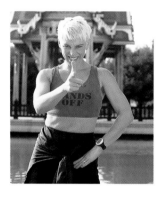

end of the day. It means having energy left over to do other things. In a nutshell, fitness is training for your heart and cardiovascular system, for muscle strength and endurance, for condition and flexibility...and of course, learning to change your eating habits over time. Fitness without proper nutrition will not help you lose those extra pounds—but it will make you stronger and more resilient and will help you at least maintain your weight.

Just last year, we began calling our aerobics classes "group fitness." A good studio offers a variety of quality cardiovascular group

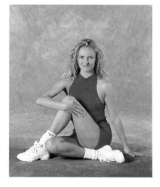

activities: low-impact, high-impact, mixed-impact, fat-burner, funk, hip-hop, step and slide, and walking. All these classes have something in common. They are the off-spring of classic aerobics.

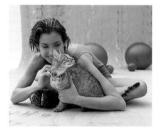

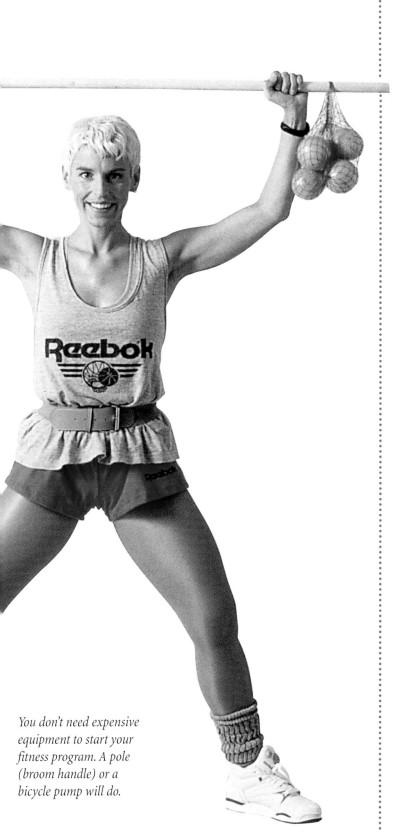

You don't need expensive equipment to start your fitness program. A pole (broom handle) or a bicycle pump will do.

a philosophy, almost a science. Instead of free-style, follow-me-if-you-can classes, we have educated instructors, music specially selected for its correct beats per minute, and aerobic research.

Better Training Results

In the late 80s, the sport shoe company Reebok was the first to declare fitness as part of its new campaign. Their new Step Reebok would stand proudly side by side with basketball, football, tennis and running. Fitness wear was born and shoes were being constructed for the aerobics followers. Aerobics branched out to mean more than just "in the presence of oxygen." Stepping, onto the adjustable platform, was created. And, to compensate for the vertical, came horizontal exercise in the form of slide. From the West Coast and New York, cardio-funk, then hip-hop classes, were born. Even stationary bike riding ("Spinning") has found its way into the aerobics classroom. Unfortunately, chronic injuries have also found their way into this euphoric training system.

Why Is Aerobics, or Group Fitness, Not Enough?

The expression "love it or leave it" applies to a lot of people who had been faithful followers of aerobics or group fitness classes. They took the classes they liked. Many started with a motivation to lose weight, others just loved the music and the endorphin high they got. If they loved step, they took every class offered. If they were high-low aerobics freaks, then you saw them in their Lycras every day, jumping up and down. Although they were having fun, their bodies were being stressed, and overuse injuries developed into chronic disorders—bad knees and spinal problems were and are still common complaints. The body that initially lost weight gained it back, and even though the amount of classroom aerobics increased, so did the weight. This is not fitness!

Suddenly, the importance of muscle training dawned on the industry. For a select few, this was no secret. Karen Voight has taught muscle strength classes for more than a decade—long before it became popular. In my club in Germany, we have had muscle-strength classes for over ten years as well. I brought weights, tubing, and rubber bands into our old "Group Fitness" classroom and taught our members about the "make-up" under the skin long before anyone dreamed of taking weights out of the body-building area.

When we first started, we called the class "Workout" and just used our own weight—a whole class working every part of our body, but without a lot of movement. Push-ups, dips, and lots of abdominal work were the beginnings. Then I was asked to act as a translator for Tammi Lee Webb, who had come to Germany to teach us how to work with rubber bands. I immediately introduced this form of resistance training into the workout.

I then convinced the club to let me buy hand weights, and with this we renamed "Workout" "Bodystyling." To this day, it is the most popular class in the club. Every bodystyling class is full, no matter what time of day. Why?

Well, it started with my models. They began working out with the rubber bands and soon saw the positive changes it made in their bodies. The women who had thought that muscle work would make them into female Arnold Schwarzeneggers were reassured that they, too, could look as lovely and defined as my models.

We soon developed a special "Abs, Glutes and Thighs" class for those special problem areas. It, too, was a major success. Now, though, our women know that all-over muscle strength is essential, and our men know that visiting a lower-body strength class is a great help in getting rid of those scrawny "chicken legs."

Back in the United States, a lot of aerobics enthusiasts had loved it...and left it! They just didn't feel so good about doing aerobics anymore; they had become disenchanted. Many switched to the fitness room, instead, and were pumping weights and using cardiovascular equipment. Those who wanted more than an endorphin high and were eager to see results booked their first one-to-one session with a personal trainer.

What Does Personal Training Offer?

Most people today know more about health and fitness then they ever did. When they make the decision to work with a personal trainer, they can chose the time that suits their schedule, they can determine where they wish to be trained—at home, in the office, in their club, at their trainer's club, outdoors or indoors. They know they are paying for the motivation that they need to achieve the goals they can't manage alone.

And a knowledgeable trainer can train them far more effectively than they could do themselves. The program is tailored to their specific needs, and not for a group of 10 to 30 people. If they follow the plan laid out for them by their trainer, and if they adjust their nutritional habits, they are almost guaranteed success in a relatively short period of time.

Each of my clients and I work out a program together. I am the guide, taking into consideration the needs, goals, lifestyle, and starting point of my client. When we train together, I observe, encourage, and correct each exercise and the movements made to effectively achieve it. I try to teach my client to move in such a way that the energy expended will have been positively applied. The client learns what technique is, and begins to understand how to bring this out in everyday life as well. I become my client's conscience. I am there to instill belief in oneself, when doubts arise. My client has the feeling that he or she is not alone.

What Exactly *Is* Personal Training?

At the same time as I developed the bodystyling and rubber band workouts for our club, a lot of members and non-members asked me if I would train them individually. I worked up tailor-made programs for them,

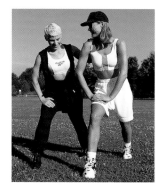

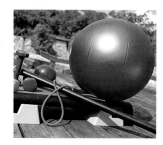

depending on their needs and lifestyles. Conditioning, strength, and flexibility were always included—it was just a matter of how much and how often. Personal training means one trainer to one client. Every person is different, even twins! Reaction to training is different, too, for each individual, even if they are similar body types. Personal training can

be implemented in many areas—from fitness, to rehabilitation, to sports. Some clients come to me because they are unhappy with their bodies. Others, because they have tried and failed every diet on the market. Some people know they need the motivation of a trainer to get started. Many who have completed physical therapy know that they cannot continue alone, and see personal training as post-rehabilitation. My clients include models, stressed-out top executives, housewives, soccer players, just about every type of person you can imagine...

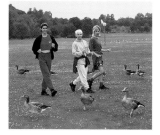

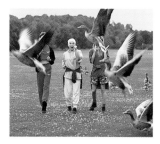

...and some you couldn't imagine!

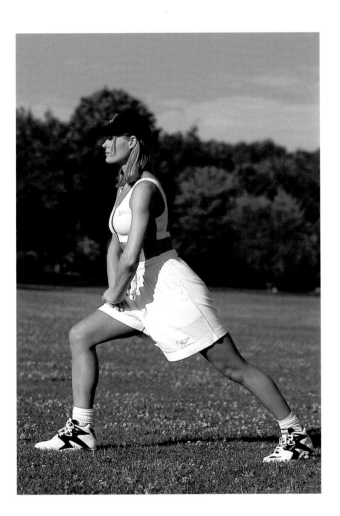

**A Versatile
Exercise Program**

Who Can Use a Personal Trainer?

Certainly those people who have tried and failed at group fitness activities and diets have need of a personal trainer. Then there are those who just don't wish to train in the public eye, such as in studios or clubs, either because they feel that they are too "unfit," over- or underweight, or uncoordinated. Then we have the very busy people, who simply come to realize that if they don't do something *now*, it's not going to happen for them. I've had so many people come to me and say, "I'm not in touch with my body." They are not overweight or overly fat; they are usually in their mid-forties, successful, and stressed out. I have helped actors, models, young mothers and grandmothers...and also post-rehab patients who know they *must* start and continue to train to achieve a healthier lifestyle, but won't do it alone.

What Does Personal Training Mean To You?

Well, first of all, with this book in hand, you have the advantage of my experience and you don't have to pay my normal fee! Now that is a bargain!

Seriously though, through this book, I will become your personal trainer and will take you where you haven't been able to go before. I want you to believe in me and in yourself, because together, with just a few changes, you will be guaranteeing yourself a better quality of life—for the rest of your life.

I have tried to put down all my experience and successes with people like you onto these pages. All the exercises have been painstakingly described and the photos carefully selected so that you can successfully follow them. If you do what I suggest, you will gain not only more physical strength and a general well-being, but you will be mentally more well-balanced and alert. You will be able to select a tailor-made program to meet your needs and goals. Start by finding your body type on pages 14–15. Go through the checklists to determine which training plan is correct for you and your lifestyle. I have tried to make understanding muscle function a little like watching "Sesame Street"— informative but fun. All the exercises are sectioned off into muscle groups. The seven lifestyle plans in the back section of the book can be combined, if your lifestyle is not completely one or another. It's not complicated—I hate complicated!

If you can discipline yourself to stick with your personal training program, I promise that you will feel and see results within six to twelve weeks. The only thing I ask of you is patience —and a smidgen of discipline!

Personal training has now become a standard practice in many clubs throughout the USA. In Germany, it is just beginning to take a foothold, although our club has offered personal training for the last 5 years!

A fitness trainer cannot give you the undivided attention of a personal trainer. Also, a personal trainer can go walking with you, an especially attractive way to train if you have a park near your club. Fresh air, anyone?

II. The First Step Is Always Hardest

One afternoon when I was picking my daughter up from her dance and musical classes, the studio owner asked me if I wanted to participate in a jazz gymnastics class. I will never, ever forget this first class, for it truly changed my life.

I stood in the front line, not in ballet tights and a leotard as in the old days, no, I had the largest sweat pants on—they were faded pink, as I recall, and were meant to hide my hips and legs. I was surrounded by ex-models, all mommies like myself—only the difference was, they still were long and trim. The mirror facing me was from ceiling to floor— not like the small mirrors at home that only revealed my narrow face and small-framed upper body. No, this was nothing like home—in front of me was a Jennifer I did not know—a living human pear! The top small and somewhat normal, the bottom huge. My legs were so fat they looked as if they were sprouting from my bottom—like a pear with feet! How could I bear to stay and move, with this vision before me? Just in time, the trainer pushed "play" on the cassette recorder and we began to move. Moving wasn't so difficult for me because of my ballet training—it was trying not to look in the mirror that became my discipline. When the class ended I felt so good. My body felt warm and energized and I was in a fantastic mood despite the nightmare in the mirror.

Normally, I would never have gone back to that class, but because of the way I felt afterwards, I decided to do something I would have never done before. I ignored the fact that I looked awful and cared more about feeling good. I couldn't wait until the next class. Pretty soon I was going a couple times a week, then every day. Moving to music in this way opened up a forgotten source of energy within me. I could feel an inner strength growing inside my body and filling my psyche. For the very first time in my life I was consistently happy! Doing something like this made life so much more worth living.

The most valuable lesson I learned from this experience, however, was to accept myself the way I was. Something I could never do before.

So I pass this on to you, my readers. Don't compare yourself with how you were 5 or 10 years ago, don't compare yourself to models or actors (who have very likely been made and not born!). Stop looking at the charts for "ideal weight," "ideal figure." Every successful fitness program must begin with you learning to love yourself...after all, even I learned to love Jennifer, the pear.

Mirror, Mirror...

It is often very difficult to accept our reflection in the mirror, especially when we continually compare ourselves to our former, younger image. This was the problem in my case. I kept hoping to greet an anorexic ballet

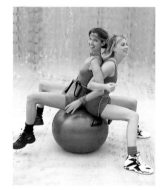

dancer, who thought she might be a top model if she grew 6 inches. My father-in-law was very athletic and even did bodybuilding as a young man. After 35, he played golf once in a great while. He complained about his ever-growing paunch and the fact that he was not as strong as he used to be. Does this sound familiar? You page

through an old photo album and think: "Wow, I really looked good then!" Only that photo is 15 years old, and you were 20 pounds lighter then, too. Don't make the mistake of constantly comparing yourself to what you once were.

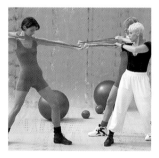

Just as your personality develops as you get older, so does your body. People can't go back to being what they used to be. But, as we mature, we can become far better looking than we ever were. It is important, however, to begin a fitness program with an open mind of how we view ourselves. Ready for change?

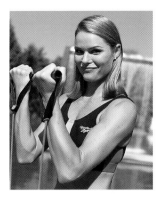

Debbie comes from Australia. Her passion is running outdoors, in nature.

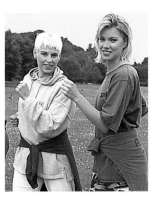

Amanda is what is known as a typical all-American girl. She loves in-line skating.

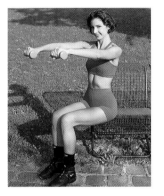

Spanish Maria trains on weights and fitness machines. She loves aerobics, too.

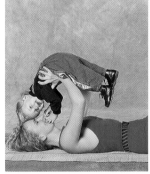

After the birth of her now 7-year-old daughter, Daniela trained herself, using videos and books!

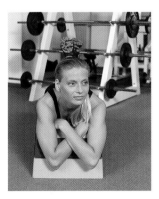

German-Danish Loren not only models but teaches aerobics and is a personal trainer.

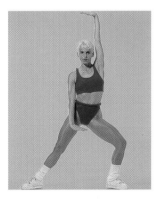

Last but not least: Jennifer's passion for fitness did not stop at step aerobics!

The Different Body Types: What Type Are You?

Are you long, lean and muscular or do you tend to gain weight easily? Are you tall, small or medium height?
Do you have a delicate frame or are you large boned?

As you analyze yourself, remember that many features are genetically predetermined. Physiologists have identified various predispositions and have categorized them into three groups: ectomorph, mesomorph, endomorph (see the table on p. 14–15). Most people are a predominate type with aspects of one or both of the others. Every person, regardless of body type, can make positive changes to their physique. Don't forget, however, that bone structure will not change, so if your hips are a little broad all the fat loss and training in the world won't make them narrow, but we can build up your upper body to even out the proportions!

You will notice that each body type has to train a little differently in order to achieve set goals. A lean, muscular person with low body fat will train differently from his/her endomorphic friend. The way you choose to train should reflect your individual needs. Let this table be a guide, reread it often if you must, and learn to train smart.

Introducing My Models: Debbie, Loren, Maria, Amanda, Daniela

Debbie is from "down under," an Australian. Her body type is primarily athletic; although her limbs are very long and lean, her lower body does tend a bit in the endomorph direction, as she gains weight "down under" very easily. She trains regularly: she's a fresh-air girl, so she loves jogging in the English Gardens in Munich. If the weather doesn't permit this, she's on the treadmill in the club, and afterwards she trains on the machines.

Our Spanish Maria has a problem everyone would love to have, especially we women. She has to remember to eat! She has long arms and legs and a delicate bone structure. We would put Maria in the ectomorph category.

The German-Danish Loren, our American Amanda, and our "Münchner Kindl" (Munich child) Daniela are real ectomorph-mesomorph types.

Loren, who is also an aerobic instructor and personal trainer, is careful to train all muscle groups, combined with a varied cardiovascular program.

With Amanda's love of tennis and skating, she doesn't find it necessary to train regularly either in a club or alone.

Daniela is the only one who is not a professional model. The mother of a seven-year-old girl, she trains regularly at home!

And me, Jennifer pear, an upper-body mesomorph and lower-body endomorph. By training smart, I have been able to build and maintain my upper body and have slowly improved and somewhat reshaped my lower body.

Body Type & Characteristics	Strength & Endurance	Sets & Reps

Ectomorph

Thin and lean, low body fat and muscle mass, high metabolism. Difficult to gain weight and increase muscle size.

Try to train at least two body parts at each workout session. Train each body part at least once per week.

Get plenty of rest between workouts: make sure the muscles have recuperated before the next session.

Change the exercise routine at least every four weeks. Try to increase the intensity at each workout.

To build muscle mass, do fewer reps; do more sets with more resistance or weights. Work your body harder for a shorter period of time. Try to train at least 3 times a week. At the start, muscle workouts have priority over cardiovascular training.

Cardiovascular exercise: walking, biking, aqua-aerobics, treadmill (walk).

Perform each exercise slowly and make sure to take enough breaks between exercises.

Do 8–12 reps, and up to 3 sets per body part.

Watch out not to overtrain, it can slow you down, causing you to lose your motivation. Overtraining can also cause problems with tendons; and muscle injuries can set you back. They could make you want to give up, so be careful!

Mesomorph

Athletic, muscular body, long torso, full chest, well-proportioned, narrow hips, broad shoulders. Builds muscles easily.

The more varied the program, the better the results.

Alternate 2 weeks of high-intensity muscle strength training with 2 to 3 weeks of lower intensity muscle endurance workouts to promote both growth and strength.

The key to your muscle workouts is variation. In this way, you avoid burn-out and overtraining.

Train at least twice a week.

Cross training is an ideal way to promote cardiovascular endurance: include walking, running, jogging, in-line skating, skiing, biking, stair climber.

Vary exercises by performing them slowly then also quickly.

The upper body can be trained with heavier weights or more resistance, the lower body with less:
Upper body: do 8–12 reps, with or without sets
Lower body: do 12–24, no sets.

Perform a whole body muscle workout once a week.

Endomorph

Big and wide bone structure, metabolism is slow, high body fat, weight gain easy because body stores fat. Muscle gain is often hidden.

Perform whole body workouts with more repetitions and less resistance and weights.

Train abdominals daily!

Avoid stairclimber and step and slide classes at first, if you tend to build legs and hips.

Frequent workouts, especially aerobic exercise (priority for fat burning): walking, biking, low-impact aerobics, cross-country skiing, treadmill (walk).

Save training in sets for later, after fat deposits are reduced.

Try to train only one set with 12–32 repetitions.

Use lighter weights and little resistance, especially when working the legs and calves.

Intensity	Recuperation	Nutrition	Lifestyle
Use heavier weights or stronger resistance to increase intensity. Rest at least one minute between sets. Train an upper body part, then train a lower body part (rest one body part, work the other). It's good for motivation and saves time. Cardiotrain in target heart rate (65–75%)	Longer recuperation time needed—take more rest days. Try to sleep 8 hours each night—especially important for those with a high metabolic rate.	Eating regularly and correctly is absolutely essential. Take supplements. Never allow yourself to go hungry. Eat snacks between main meals. Ideal: 5–7 small meals per day. If building muscle mass, include weight gain drinks. Protein intake 25–30%. Carbohydrates 50%. Fats 20–25%. Drink plenty of liquids. Try to take in 10 glasses (8 oz. per glass) of water per day. Drink a protein shake 1½–2 hours before going to bed,	Try to keep stress levels in check by learning how to relax. (Tip: Try Yoga, Meditation, Tai-Chi.) Conserve energy by eliminating unnecessary activity. In all that you do, think energy conservation.
Variation is the key to success: increase and decrease intensity with exercises, sets, reps, weights and rest—this is valid for both muscle and cardio training. Use full range of motion and alternate reps by working slowly, then with moderate, then with fast pace. Cardiotrain in target heart rate (65–75%).	Proper rest is essential to enhance and then maintain your natural advantage. Average 7 (5–9) hours of sleep. Make sure that the trained body part is fully recovered before you renew training.	Protein intake should equal 1 gram per pound of body weight Carbohydrate intake should be relatively high: 60% of total calorie intake. Limit fats: 10–20%. Drink 10 8-oz. glasses of water per day.	Too much too fast is a no-no! Injuries, over training and burnout could result (muscles and tendons are susceptible and at risk). Patience and discipline are necessary to reach and maintain goals. Your motto: Slow down and listen to your body.
If sets are performed , keep intensity high—no more than 60 seconds rest between them. Cardiotrain in the lower level of your target heart rate (55–65%). Start program slowly and build up to working longer and harder. Don't overdo—especially if you have been a long-time couch potato!	Train frequently Cardiotrain daily if time allows. For muscle training, allow 48 hours between exercises of the same body part. Because of a slower metabolism you won't need as much sleep. 7.5 hours is recommended.	Keep fat intake low (under 20%). Consume dairy products that are non-fat (eliminate cheeses). Eat smaller meals more often to keep blood sugar levels up and to control appetite—but control snacking. Avoid late night eating. Say no to second helpings. Eliminate soft drinks and alcohol. Try to drink at least 10 8-oz. glasses of water per day. Think of your calorie consumption as a bank account!	Try to include more aerobic activities in your daily routine. Ride your bike to work. Park your car farther away from work or school. Climb the stairs instead of taking an elevator or escalator, and *walk, walk, walk!* Keep yourself moving! Use as much energy in your daily life as possible. Run your own errands instead of sending someone. Even stand up and sit down more often! Every movement counts!

General Training Guidelines

● **Training** Depending on how much time you can invest in your training and what body type you are, you can do one set for every body part or you can do more sets and concentrate on one or two body parts. If you plan to train two body parts, for example, try to train agonist and antagonist (negative and positive). You could train one upper body part and one lower.

● **Muscle Strength and Cardiovascular Endurance** Muscle strength will help you lift boxes and take care of heavy loads. Muscle endurance will help you be able to repeat a movement many times without tiring. Muscle workouts will tone, define or build, depending on the type of training you chose. Cardiovascular endurance will develop the heart and lungs so they will function more efficiently and stay healthy into very old age. Low intensity cardiovascular workouts are good for everybody — from fat burning for those wishing to lose body fat to those well-trained "toughies" who have to regenerate their overworked systems.

● **Repetitions and Sets** Repetitions, or reps, are the amount of times you do a single movement in an exercise. You bend your arm 8 times (bicep curl)—you have done 8 reps. If you do 8 reps, take a 30-second break, then do 8 more bicep curls, you have done 2 sets of 8 reps! Sets are groups of reps!

● **Intensity** In muscle training, intensity is how much weight or resistance you use. In cardiovascular training, the intensity is measured by your heart rate. The best way to actually see your heart rate is by wearing a heart rate monitor.

● **Recuperation** Rest periods are absolutely essential to success in fitness. Whether it's the 60-second break between sets or the 24 to 48 hours between training sessions, your muscles need time to regenerate. It is during this regeneration period that the muscles become even stronger. This is the principle of "supercompensation." It is only through properly dosed rest between exercises or days of exercises that gains in strength and/or endurance are achieved.

● **Nutrition** Good eating habits are the main key to achieving the best, quickest and most long lasting results. See my tips starting on page 142.

● **Lifestyle** Our mode of living must slowly change to a healthy way of living. Everything that we do in the training room has to be carried over to our everyday and working lives. It is called "making choices"! Learning to distinguish between indulgence and nutrition starts with drinking water or sipping herbal flavored teas to quench thirst instead of downing a cold soda! Beer and soft drinks are indulgences and can be enjoyed as such, but water is something our bodies and organs need to stay healthy!

Target Heart Rate

Your heart rate is the rate at which your heart beats per minute. During any training exercise or movement, sport physiologists recommend a so-called target heart rate, which is calculated from an estimated maximum heart rate of 220 minus your age. Target heart rates range 60–75% less than the maximum rate. Your own target rate depends on your age and physical condition. For an exact measurement, determine your resting (lowest) heart rate—on waking from sleep. Your target rate is also determined by the length of your training unit. If you train longer than 30 minutes, you will want to train at a lower heart rate. The older you are, the lower your range will be.

Average Target Heart Rate		
Age	Target Range (60–75%)	Maximum Heart Rate (220 less age)
20	120–150	200
25	117–146	195
30	114–142	190
35	111–138	185
40	108–135	180
45	105–131	175
50	102–127	170
55	99–123	165
60	96–120	160
65	93–116	155
70	90–113	150

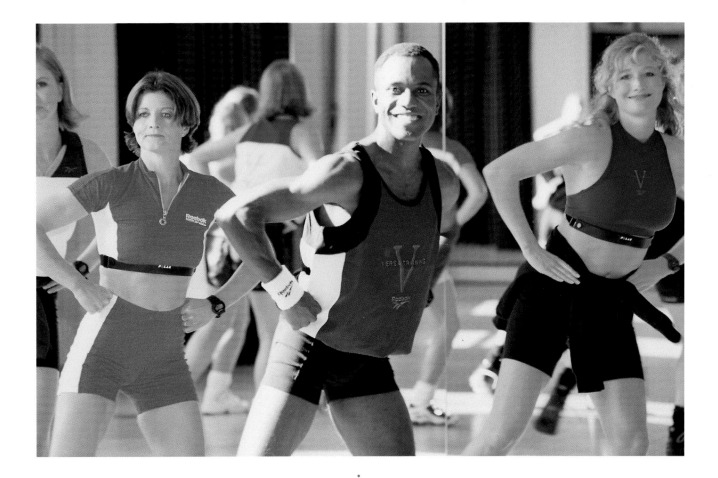

Exercising to music in a group can be very motivating.

Training Tips

Start out slowly and gradually increase your training frequency, time and intensity. Doing too much too soon is a sure way of getting burned out fast, injuring yourself, becoming unmotivated! If you haven't exercised before or in a long time (no matter how active you were before), consult a doctor before embarking on an exercise program. A sports medicine specialist can work out your proper training level.

What Exactly *Is* Your Lifestyle?

Apart from your body type, the second most important factor in constructing a successful training program is the way you live. If your fitness program is also going to improve the quality of your life, we have to examine more closely your daily living habits and the circumstances under which you live.

I take a lot of time interviewing my prospective clients. I not only feel a need to medically screen them, but to find out the different aspects of their lives in order for me to conceive and work out an absolutely individual and effective training program for them.

You, my readers, since I am not *actually* there with you, must do this part of my job for me. In order to accomplish this, I have prepared a checklist about living habits, working habits, and an assessment of yourself as a beginner or advanced exerciser. This information will help you to determine which plan is the most effective for you.

By using the checklist and the information provided, you will also become aware of risk factors and how they relate to certain diseases. It will cover the effects of nicotine, alcohol, medication, etc., as well as unhealthy eating habits and chronic fatigue.

Let's Look at Your Working Environment

Are you forced to sit a lot of the time?

Then the "Office Prisoners" training plan (p. 128) is the right one for you. This plan has been worked up specifically to help all those who spend most of their working hours sitting at a desk and/or working on a computer.

Sitting for hours on end weakens our trunk muscles, i.e. the back and stomach muscles. The chest and hip flexor muscles are usually very tight. If you have problems with your knees anyway, then marathon sitting sessions will aggravate the problem even more. Almost everyone I know who works in an office environment has bad posture and lower back discomfort. You will find the perfect plan to help free you from all these muscular imbalances. The exercises are easy and require no more space than a chair!

Office Prisoners need to escape—so I also highly recommend beginning an aerobic exercise program to complete your quest for freedom.

Do you stand for most of the day?

If you're a hairdresser, a cameraman, or a dentist, you've likely been heard to complain about your swollen and aching legs and feet. Some of you, if you're genetically predisposed, will have varicose veins, aggravated by constant standing. Your normal leg activity becomes static if you stand in one place for a long time. Because of this, the auxiliary "muscle pump" function of the legs becomes limited. Healthy active legs aid the body in circulating blood and lymph fluids. As the muscles are not being contracted, the fluids are not being transported, hence the swelling in our extremities.

The trunk muscles have to help keep us erect the whole day, so the back will be tense. You're probably holding your arms in front of you to accomplish your tasks, so you will have sore shoulders and your chest muscles will be very tight. Usually, my clients who work in the standing professions also have bad pos-ture. The upper back is usually growing into a fine little hump!

My plan "Standing for Hours" is your guide to a strong trunk and healthy legs that will swell no more. And, the little hump in your upper back will magically disappear! Turn to page 130.

Does your job require you to travel all the time?

If you're always on the road, it's *impossible* to find the time and place to do anything involved with fitness, right? I say, "On the Go? No Excuses!" Here's a plan for anywhere, anytime (p. 132).

I'll help you learn to use those free moments between appointments or when you are in your hotel room. Use the stairs instead of the elevator or escalator. Walk to the taxi-stand instead of having the taxi pick you up. Encourage your business partner to

What's Your Sex?

Male/female? The training programs that I have designed are for both men and women. Because you men were blessed with more strength than we females, I encourage you male readers to work with heavier weights and stronger tubing...but *only* after you have acquired impeccable technique!

How Fit Do You Think You Are?

How old are you?
15–20
21–30
31–40
41–50
51 or older?

No matter your age, if you are embarking on your first fitness experience, follow all the recommendations for beginners.
You should train all body parts, even if you think you only need to exercise triceps and adductors.

Remember, also, how important it is to do a proper warm-up. Your joints and muscles will thank you afterwards. As we grow older, we lose flexibility and elasticity. Take this into consideration and warm up accordingly. If you do the exercises on a regular basis, you will soon see progress, and after only four to six weeks, you can advance to the next fitness level.

What's Your "At Work" Schedule?

Are your working hours regular? 9:00 a.m. to 5:00 a.m.? Or irregular, because you travel or work different shifts? If up to now you've made excuses because of having to work irregular hours, turn to page 132. You'll have "No Excuses" anymore, because I have exercises "to go"— so you can't say no!

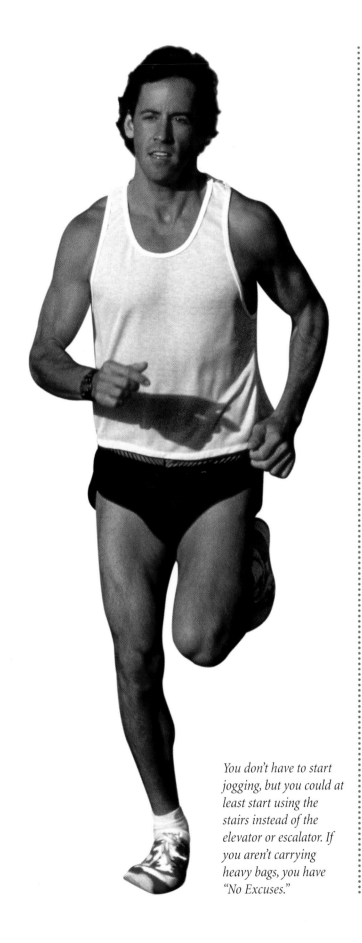

You don't have to start jogging, but you could at least start using the stairs instead of the elevator or escalator. If you aren't carrying heavy bags, you have "No Excuses."

go for a walk after that filling executive lunch. It's a great way to discuss your next deal.

I have simple but effective exercises for all body parts that can be performed in your hotel, in a plane, in a train, even in your car! You can start today—just turn to page 132!

Do you have a physically active job?

Depending on what you do, you may be one of the lucky ones! If you are a real sports "jock," a fanatic fitness freak, or your job requires lots of manual labor, you have a plus in the cardiovascular department. Your problems probably lie in the onesidedness of your activities. If you play tennis, one arm will always be stronger and even larger than the other. A horseback rider or soccer player will have very tight inner thigh muscles. If you work as a nurse and must lift people all the time, then your back is being stressed many hours on end.

If I had you in front of me, I could tell you exactly what we could do. Instead, you, my readers, must determine your stress points, then use my special plan for "Toughies" on page 134.

How Do You Spend Your Leisure Time?

Friends and family

How about bringing those friends and family into your active fitness program? If it hadn't been for my very best friend Camille, I wouldn't have had the courage to go running at 5:30 a.m. when I was a teenager. Now that's a friend!

You new moms out there can certainly use such support. Put the little ones down for a nap and start my "Models and New Moms" program (p. 136). If your kids are older, combine the program with "Hip Hop Kids" (p. 138). My shaping-up program includes exercises to help tone the muscles of the hips, buttocks and thighs—teen Hip Hop girls will join Mom for sure.

A little something about *cellulite:* In Europe as in America, women are plagued with wads of cellulite. In much American fitness literature, cellulite is brushed off in a sentence or two as merely "fat." In Europe, especially France and Germany, univer-sities have done extensive studies on cellulite. Some studies go back to 1816, when Balfour first commented on the coetaneous nodule formations later named cellulite. In-depth German and Italian studies, comparing cellulite to normal fat, concluded that cellulite is, indeed, a specific syndrome—see page 20.

Cellulite doesn't just occur in the overweight; there are many women with *peau d'orange* who have no weight problems. We know that those suffering from cellulite have a genetic predisposition to this problem. Environmental pollution, junk food, coffee and tea, additives, hormonal changes and disturbances can all encourage this syndrome. During pregnancy, it is quite natural to develop cellulite on the hips.

Cellulite vs. Fat

This is cellulite:

- a leakage of plasma through weakened capillary walls into the spaces between fat cells
- a thickening of connective fiber which encapsulates fat cells
- nodule formation caused by the hardening of collagen
- a stretching of capillaries, and blood-and-lymph stagnation from poor circulation

Helpful tips to fight cellulite:

- drink plenty of water
- avoid impact exercises
- eat lots of fiber and nutrient-rich fruits and vegetables
- stop smoking

I have learned a secret in training my female clients who have cellulite problems. Because the cell tissue of those suffering from cellulite is very soft and weak, I encourage my clients to practice such non-impact cardiovascular-endurance exercises, as walking, stepping (no jumping!), biking, swimming or aqua-aerobics (especially good!). Eating properly, detoxifying the system, and lymph-drainage massages are all helpful in the cellulite war!

Playing sports

If you like to play sports, turn to page 134. I put this plan together especially for the athletic type. When I take on an athlete as a personal training client, I work with him, or her, on an entirely different basis to that which he is accustomed. I am not training him for his special skill. I leave that up to his coach. I work on all the imbalances that have developed because of the one-sidedness of the sport. Usually, my "toughies" have many old injuries that cause many other problems. Because exercise and sport is specific, I challenge them with new activities that require grace, a different kind of coordination and balance. Muscles that are tight will be stretched, weak muscles will be strengthened. If you have ever seen a football player take a simple step-aerobics class, you would wonder how they can play their game so well! But, with practice and patience, I have made a good "stepper" out of the most uncoordinated linebacker!

I was very fit as a ballet dancer, but I was the worst athlete imaginable. I was thrown from horses, totally out of control on the ski slopes, and a miserable iceskater. When I was very young and we had to do the 50-yard dash, the other kids would laugh at me, saying I looked like a penguin running!

How to Burn Off Fat

If you want to burn fat, you should train in a 3-to-2 ratio of cardio and muscle; that means three times a week you should be performing some aerobic activity.

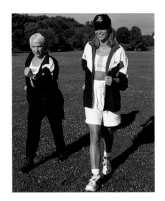 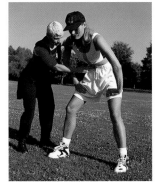

In order to stimulate the metabolism to burn fat, it is important to chose a form of exercise that you can carry out longer, but that is of low to middle intensity. I know what I'm talking about. In 1993, my very longest and most hard working personal training client, who in the beginning was probably one of the weakest and most uncoordinated, developed a passion for walking. She booked me three to four times a week and we walked miles and hours through the English Gardens in Munich. In the beginning, her walking was as slow as a snail and her technique needed constant correction, but after several weeks, she developed into a great walker with a good level of intensity. Meanwhile, without having changed anything else in my life or working schedule, I had lost almost 10 pounds! So it was after that summer of low-intensity walking that my theoretical knowledge was confirmed by my own reaction to this form of training. I encourage all my clients and students to adopt the motto "light is right" if they want to burn fat.

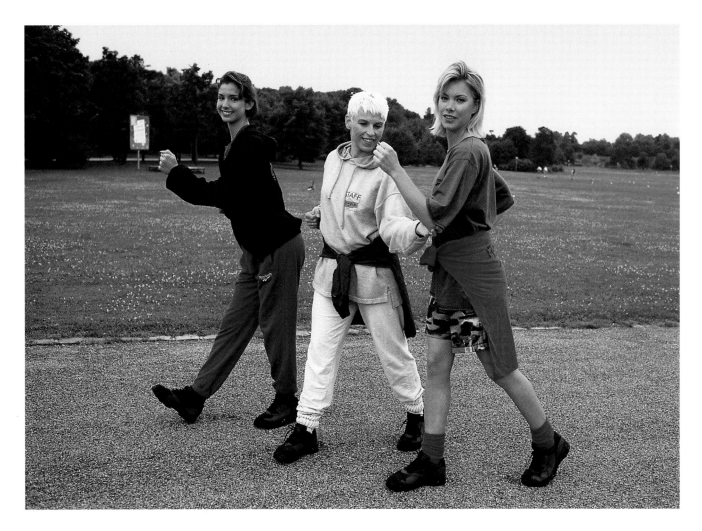

That Simple but Marvelous Exercise: Walking!

Most people nowadays are not surprised to hear that moderate walking has proven to reduce health risks and prolong life and to increase cardio-vascular endurance over a longer period of time. But walking also relieves stress and serves as a perfect recuperative activity to other more intensive sport activities.

For people who have trouble with coordination, walking is an especially good exercise. It helps to consciously get arms and legs working in sync. Because of the pace, walking allows you to really work on your posture and technique. Isn't it amazing that something so simple and everyday can be so effective!

Some words here about muscular imbalance: Personal training is particularly good for helping people become aware of their muscular imbalances. They learn not only the appropriate exercises as a remedy for these problems, but become aware of what causes these imbalances. All muscles have partners! We call them agonists and antagonists. When one muscle stretches, the other bends. Just like a pulley, both partners must possess the right amount of tension or strength. If one side is too strong or tight, this interferes with proper muscle function. It causes discomfort and even, eventually, leads to injury. If you train only your bicep muscles, your triceps will atrophy and any movements involving the tricep muscle (like pushing yourself upwards with your arms) will be very difficult.

I already mentioned the problem with tennis players. If you compare their playing arm with their other arm, the circumference of the playing arm greatly exceeds the other. If you didn't know they played tennis, you might think the non-playing arm is just out of a cast! If the other arm isn't trained as well, shoulder and trunk tightness can result.

Squash players stress their knees constantly by the sudden stops and turns they make on the court. If they train the muscles around their knees correctly, they can play squash for years to come without suffering knee discomfort or injury.

Horseback riders must make concerted efforts to train abductor muscles to offset shortened and tight adductors (inner thigh).

A little tip: Think about which muscles you use most when playing your favorite sport. Look at the exercises offered and put a program together for yourself. Is your lower body stronger and larger in proportion to your upper body? Where do your muscular weaknesses lie? For sure there are exercises made to order for you; just turn to the "Toughie" chapter.

In front of the TV

Hello, Couch Potato! I know what you're about to say. You've had a hard day. Totally stressed out from work, you have carry-out on your lap and a cold drink nearby to wash it down. Some taco chips and dip are handy, in case you get hungry again. Here, on the couch, you are lulled into a heavenly snooze, until you suddenly wake up and find it's time to go to bed!

The only muscles a couch potato might develop are the biceps, repeatedly bringing food to the mouth. Oh yes, the jaw muscles, from chewing, and the overused thumb or finger muscles from channel hopping. But seriously, how many times a week does the above scene happen? If you tell me at least three times a week, and you aren't doing any regular physical activity other than just getting up and going to work...it's time to turn to page 140. Let's do something for your health. The most important rule for you, however, is to *take things slow*. I hate the cliché, but Rome really wasn't built in a day, nor was New York City, and certainly not a body like Arnold Schwarzenegger's...but we don't want to build up that much, do we!

Start by trying to change one thing at a time. If you can just force yourself, in the beginning, to train once or twice a week, it will be an enormous step toward the first stages of fitness for you. If you are consistent and increase your training to three days a week, you will see some positive changes within twelve weeks.

Start with walking just 10 minutes a day and doing the Couch Potato exercises once or twice a week. I promise you, it will help!

As you review your work and leisure habits you can identify some warning signs: too much sitting, too little sleep, work hours inordinately long, not enough oxygen in the workplace, too many business trips. Try to ascertain which things you can change and how you can change them. For the things you cannot change, there are alternative measures. One is training to be fit. If you don't, you risk developing chronic ailments which can cause you to lose motivation and can lead to total burnout.

I need not mention the other issues which influence our lives. These are the emotional and social pressures, like stress in our work or in our relationships. Media and society say, "Take a Prozac and forget it!" It's easy, but not always the answer. It's often better to go the natural way. There's a saying, everywhere, about "a sound mind in a sound body." I like that expression!

Examining Your Eating and Drinking Habits

Experts maintain that nutrition contributes 75% to the state of our health. I believe that figure is conservative. How, what and when we feed ourselves determines so much of our whole constitution. Just think, if you put a diet cola into your gas tank, your car wouldn't run, now, would it?

If you take an honest look at your eating habits, they might

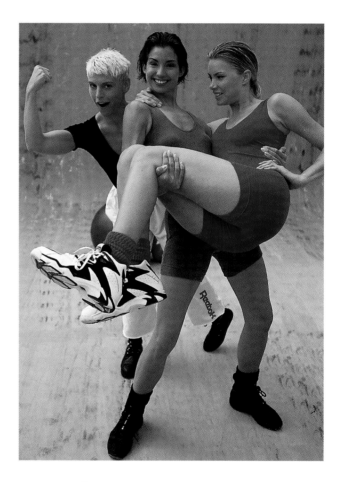

Come on, give yourself a little kick in the pants, and get off the couch! It's time you did something positive for yourself. You'll soon see results that will make you proud. One word of wisdom: Put together a program for yourself that you can have fun with, otherwise it will be just another obligation (a *should* instead of a *want*) and you'll soon start tiring of the "chore" and end up dropping out.

Assess Yourself!

How do you feel about yourself?
- ☐ overweight
- ☐ underweight
- ☐ normal weight

Why do you think you are this way?
- ☐ too many calories per day
- ☐ too few calories per day
- ☐ too much fat
- ☐ too many sweets
- ☐ too much alcohol
- ☐ genetics
- ☐ sedentary lifestyle

What are your eating habits?
- ☐ I eat regular meals
- ☐ I always eat irregularly
- ☐ I eat my main meal late at night
- ☐ I drink a lot of liquids
- ☐ I don't drink enough liquids
- ☐ I drink a lot of alcohol
- ☐ I hardly ever drink alcohol

Read my chapter on Nutrition (p. 142) and my tips for you, then come back to this little questionnaire and reassess your habits.

Do you drink alcohol every day, several times a day, or more than 4 to 8 oz. a day?
- ☐ never
- ☐ seldom
- ☐ often

Do you smoke?
- ☐ no
- ☐ yes
  - **If yes, how many cigarettes per day?** ____

What is your current fitness status?
- ☐ not so fit
- ☐ fit
- ☐ regular exerciser

show you why you are overweight or overly fat (overly fat doesn't necessarily mean overweight). Does it come from bad eating habits at work, just because you love fast food, or love it on the sweet side? Are fatty foods your downfall, or you drink a lot of alcohol? Maybe it's that you are a totally sedentary person and don't burn it up; or it's a combination of everything.

When I interview clients, I ask them to bring me a 3-day list of what and when they eat. It includes two days during the week and one day on the weekend. Normally, they are very honest, because they *want* to reach their goals. We discuss their 3-day plan and determine together where to make positive changes.

I do not believe in diets. In 1978, Covert Bailey wrote, in his first edition of *Fit or Fat,* that "diets make you fat." I not only believe that, I *know* it! I fought with the diet syndrome for years. I just wish I had read his book in 1978! If you have an eating disorder, or you suspect you have one, I urge you to seek professional help. I know what it is like to suffer from anorexia. My suggestions here for eating healthfully can be taken into consideration when the emotional eating problem has been brought under control first.

I don't need to spend time here on the dangers of nicotine and alcohol. Americans are well aware of the dangers of both. Passive smoking, especially, has become a major issue. As a vehement non-smoker, I hope that the good example set by the American Surgeon General will catch on here in Germany. Nicotine not only causes lung cancer and heart disease, but cardiovascular endurance also suffers from the smoking habit. Alcohol, if abused, is a drug that can be as lethal as heroin—and it also makes you put on fat!

Where Are You on the Fitness Scale?

Fill in the fitness checklist item on the left. Where do you think you stand? If you feel you're a beginner, stick to the guidelines for beginners when doing the exercises.

If you're not sure where you fit on the scale, read on. To determine your *exact* fitness level, you can visit a good fitness center that does fitness testing. The very famous Dr. Kenneth Cooper Institute for Aerobic Research in Dallas, Texas, is the ultimate in fitness testing. Some universities carry out fitness testing in their sports departments.

When very well-trained persons come to me, I do tests to determine their level. They are already motivated and are familiar with the concept of training. As a rule, though, I do not test people because, in the beginning, the tests only serve to depress my clients. It only confirms what they already know. I feel the first session must bring success and a feeling of fun. As I work with people, I can then determine how flexible they are, where they have the most muscle tightness. I always start with walking and light-intensity exercises, and can determine cardiovascular strength because I have all my clients wear heart rate monitors. By watching their movements, I can see how coordinated the clients are, how much balance they have.

Because I am not personally there to guide you, the exercises here will help you get to know your body. You must start out conservatively and, as you feel the strength growing within, you may accordingly vary or increase your intensity.

The following flexibility and cardio tests are for you to use to judge yourself, because I am not there to do them. If you go through the results of the tests and answer the checklist objectively, you will be able to determine your beginning level.

Shoulder Girdle Flexibility Test

Put both hands behind your back, one arm raised and bent so you are touching your hand to your shoulder blade. Take the other arm behind your waist and try to touch the bottom of your shoulder blade.
● If you are able to grasp your hands together behind your back, you have normal flexibility in the shoulder girdle.
● If you can only bring the tips of the fingers together, you should try to improve your range of motion. That means start stretching regularly.
● If you cannot even bring your fingertips together, you are extremely tight. You must do as much stretching as possible.

Heart Rate Recovery: A 3-Minute Step Test

Warm up sufficiently before you begin this test (see warm-ups, page 126), then check your pulse before you start.
● **Starting position:** Stand near a step platform or use stairs. The platform height should be about 8 (beginner), 10 (average) or 12 (advanced) inches. Keep the back straight, the knees soft and the stomach muscles pulled together You can let the arms hang loosely at your sides, or place your hands on your hips.
● **Exercise:** Starting with your left foot, step up onto the platform, bring the right foot up, then step down with the left foot and then the right. Step up and down as fast as you can for one minute starting left, then without stopping change to your right foot and step up starting with the right foot. Do this for one minute. For the last minute, you can step either with the right or left (so altogether you've stepped 3 minutes without stopping).
● **Evaluation:** Sit down quickly and measure your pulse for one minute. After a minute, you will have your recovery heart rate.
● **Warning:** If you are at all dizzy, feel faint or are short of breath during this test, stop immediately!
● **Tip:** When stepping, place the heel on the step first and roll onto the balls of the feet. When stepping down, roll from the toes to the heels. The heels remain on the floor and do not bounce or jiggle up and down. Try to stay close to the platform and stand erect, not leaning forward or backward.

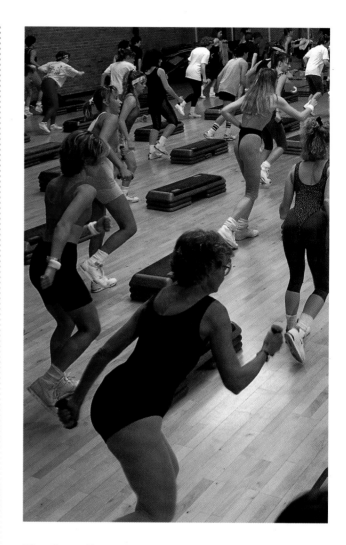

The Step Test

Before proceeding with the step test, you must do the following:
● **Warm up sufficiently (6 minutes' time or so would be good).**
● **Don't choose the 12-inch platform if you are a newcomer or have been inactive for a long time.**
● **Know that it's normal to get out of breath a** little when stepping, but should you have actual shortness of breath, stop immediately!
Remember, this is only a test and you are not in a fitness center. So, if you have problems with this part of the testing, just test your flexibility and we'll concentrate on walking as your cardio-vascular exercise!

Body composition

The first thing I tell my clients is to throw away the bathroom scales. For many of us, our day is determined by the numbers we see boldly glaring up at us.

The weight registering on the scale is only telling you part of the story. Two people of the same sex, height and weight will look entirely different. One will turn heads because of an attractive figure, while the other will wear big baggy clothes to hide a "jelly roll"!

Even though Covert Baily told us about this in 1978, most people still don't understand that it is the relationship of body fat to body mass (muscles, tendons, ligaments, bones) that determines not only our state of health but also our appearance. These two factors, plus the amount of water in our body, gives us the weight we read on our bathroom scales. When we speak of body fat, we mean not only the fat directly under our skin, but the fat that lies in and around our muscles and organs.

Generally, 27% body fat is normal for a woman and 23% is normal for a man. As your fitness status improves, your body fat level should go down. There are various methods of measuring body fat. The simplest is taking skinfold measurements. The trainer measures various body sites with a skinfold caliper. This measurement, of course, cannot tell you much about your organic fat. A more comprehensive method is either hydrostatic (underwater) testing, which is very expensive, or infrared, using a device that sends a harmless electrical impulse through the body. If you are interested in finding out more about your body composition, ask about it in a good fitness center near you.

The Optimal Heart Rate

If your heart rate is abnormally high, I recommend having your doctor give you a EKG Stress Test before you begin any exercise program. If your range is average to good, you can start my exercise program in the beginner category. And if your results are excellent, you can jump into the advanced level.

Heart Rate per Minute in Recovery

Male

Age	average	fair–good	excellent
20–29	102+	100–76	74-
30–39	102+	100–80	78-
40–49	106+	104–82	80-
50+	106+	104–84	82-

Female

Age	average	fair–good	excellent
20–29	112+	110–88	86-
30–39	114+	112–88	86-
40–49	116+	114 –90	88-
50+	118+	116–92	90-

+ this figure and higher
– this figure and lower

Blood pressure and resting heart rate

Blood pressure is the force that moves blood through the circulatory system. Systolic pressure (the top number) represents the force of the blood against the walls of the arteries during the heart's contraction. Diastolic pressure (the bottom number) is the force of the blood against the artery walls when the heart is between beats.

A blood pressure reading of 120/80 while at rest is usual for an adult. Readings slightly higher than 120/80 are also acceptable. Readings as low as 90/60 are not uncommon for young women. Readings above 140/90 are considered high and, if you get this reading, check your pressure again a few minutes later.

There are many good digital blood pressure machines on the market. It might be a good idea to have one at home. However, they do not replace the competency of a doctor, and should be checked out for accuracy by your own physician.

Heart rates: resting/training/recovery

You can measure your pulse, or heart rate, very easily. Place your first two fingers (never the thumb!) either on your wrist in line with with your thumb (your radial artery), or on your neck, right or left of your Adam's apple and up slightly (your carotid artery) —don't press too hard. Do you feel the pulse? OK, now count how many times it pulses in 10 seconds. Multiply that number by six and you will have your heart rate per minute.

It's often difficult to detect and count your pulse during a training session. I encourage my clients to invest in a heart-rate monitor—a lightweight band worn around the chest with a watch on the wrist. This way, you can easily monitor your heart during all training activities, and assess your training heart rate over a period of time.

To determine resting heart rate, take your pulse in the morning upon waking up. Rates between 60–80 beats per minute are considered average. Top athletes often have resting pulses of 36 beats per minute and under!

If you are fit, you will recuperate far more quickly after exercising than someone who is not in condition. Your pulse will return to its starting point far faster. The harder you work, the higher your pulse will climb. Turn to my chapter on cardiovascular training starting on page 118.

By now you've assessed your lifestyle and your current fitness status. In order for us to create the perfect plan for you, you and I need to know what your fitness goals are.

What are your fitness goals?

Read through the list to your right and decide which priorities you wish to set for your training goals. Whatever you choose, remember that our muscle program is the starting point and basis for everything else.

● **Tip:** Remember, fitness is much more than just losing weight or looking attractive. Being fit will fill your life with new vitality, energy and power, which in turn can change many things in your life. Looking good is a side-effect—that which you have within will radiate outward.

General Exercise Recommendations

Intensity

When doing muscle strength and muscle endurance exercises, start with light weights and resistance. Only increase the intensity when your muscles are no longer fatigued after the given reps and sets. It is far more important to maintain proper technique when carrying out an exercise. In this way, you insure that the muscle is being trained correctly and efficiently. I have already mentioned how to calculate your target heart rate for exercising cardiovascularly, but just in case, let's review: 220 minus your age equals your maximal heart rate.

● **Training ranges for fat burning (and speeding up metabolism):** Take your maximal heart rate and multiply it by 50%—this will be your lower range for exercising. Now multiply your maximal heart rate by 65% for your upper range for exercising. Try to stay within these ranges when training aerobically.

● **Training ranges for improving cardiorespiratory endurance:** Multiply your maximal heart rate by 65% for your lower range, and 75% for your upper range. These ranges are more intense and will help you on the way to more cardiovascular and cardiorespiratory endurance.

Recuperation

Always leave one day between training the same body parts. The abdominals and the muscles around your knee are an exception. They can be trained daily, especially if you have back or knee problems. I recommend exercise 1 on page 83, and 7 on page 86, for the abdominals, exercise 6 on page 79 for your back and, for

Your Personal Fitness Goals

☐ **I want to gain weight.**
You should center on muscle strength training.

☐ **I would like to lose body fat.**
You should center on cardiovascular endurance training.

☐ **I want to get fit and have more energy and strength in my everyday life.**
You should do both muscle strength and cardiovascular exercise in equal amounts.

☐ **I'm a regular exerciser, I play a particular sport in my spare time, I'm an athlete centering on one major sport activity. I need a balanced program to compensate for my other training activities.**
I recommend complete body training. It is important to work on all the muscle groups, especially those neglected by your sports training. Your cardiovascular component should be regenerative if your main training is cardio intense. If your other training has little cardio work, then you should perform crosstraining activities.

☐ **I just had a baby and want to get back in shape.**
First, get a clearance from your physician. Then, concentrate on strengthening your trunk, i.e., upper and lower back, gluteal and abdominal muscles. Don't neglect your arms and shoulders.

☐ **I've just gone through physical therapy and want to get totally fit.**
You will need a special program that should first be discussed with your doctor and physical therapist.

☐ **I'd like to improve my mobility (range of motion) and flexibility. I'm so stiff and tense most of the time.**
Start with the exercises for stretching, read the section on breathing very closely and incorporate exercises for the lower back and abdominals into your daily life.

☐ **Sorry, but I'm none of the above.**
If the other statements above don't apply to you and your problems, I suggest a balanced program of all-over muscle training and regular cardiovascular exercise that is compatible with your lifestyle.

Before you can kick up your heels and yell, "I did it!" —you're going to have to put some effort into this program. Personal training offers you the possibility of developing your own program— no recipes meant for the masses—you are the one that matters. Your own program is as adjustable as this step!

your knees, turn to page 99, exercises 1 and 2. If you can manage it, you can do these exercises daily. The leg extensions can be done freely and are particularly good for "Office Prisoners."

You can perform light cardiovascular exercise daily. Heavy-duty cardiovascular exercise demands rest days as well, or can be alternated with regenerative cardio exercise in between: walking, for example.

Length and frequency of exercise

Muscle workouts three times a week and cardio four times would be optimal, for example. You can train as long as it takes you to finish your exercise plan for that day. Unfortunately, very few of you have that much time. So why not do a little every day; 10 minutes a day is a start.

You could do biceps/triceps on Monday morning, quadriceps/hamstrings on Tuesday morning, chest/upper back on Wednesday morning, and so on. Why not do a small set of abdominals every evening an hour or two before you go to bed? Stretching can be done in front of the TV set—perfect for the ex-Couch Potato! And remember, a little exercise is far better than nothing at all. The main thing is not to give up!

Special Exercise Tips

Tips for toughies

According to exercise physiologists, if you are relatively fit and train only once a week at the same level each time, you will be able to maintain that level, but will not make improvements. For you advanced exercisers and athletes who tend to do the sport, attend the exercise class or use the same cardio machine you love, but notice that you are not progressing in your training or your body is not shaping up to what you want it to be, I recommend cross training (see page 121).

Tips for training after pregnancy

Before starting or re-entering a fitness program, consult your doctor. I always ask my post-partum clients for a clearance from their gynecologist. Abdominals and back muscles will usually take precedence in the beginning phases. Of course, chest and shoulders are very important, too—for carrying the baby for the next few months…and years. Babies, by the way, are great "variable resistance"—ever-increasing weight! If you have gained extra fat during the pregnancy, then fat-burning sessions are in order. Also, no-impact exercises—aqua-aerobics and walking are great. Biking could be a little uncomfortable so soon after giving birth, but if you have no problems with it you can join a "spinning" class or get on that home stationary bike—or you can put the baby in a special carrier on your back and bike everywhere. (Just take *every* safety precaution, and watch the traffic, please!)

Post-rehabilitation

More and more people are turning to personal trainers after going through rehab with physical therapists. If you have just finished such sessions, consult with your therapist, or your doctor, before embarking on a program. Perhaps, if you show them this book, they might be able to help you make selections according to your special needs.

Important: Be patient with yourself and don't overdo. In the first phase of training, my recommendation for everyone is to simply *walk*—slow and easy for the out-of-shape and those seeking recuperative benefits, and fast and athletic for our toughies.

Training Apparel and Equipment

One of the things my new clients and I discuss before the first training session is appropriate training wear and equipment. In choosing clothing, two things are important: comfort and breatheability.

You must feel comfortable in what you have on. This means you have the freedom of movement you need to train well and you can bear to look at yourself in the mirror. (The color suits you and the pants are long or wide enough to cover what you'd rather not see—yet!) The material must "breathe" and absorb or disperse perspiration to regulate body temperature. Also, you shouldn't dress too warmly. I recommend dressing like an onion. By dressing *in layers*, you can peel off something as body and air temperatures demand: tights under sweat pants and a T-shirt under a sweat shirt are great!

Shoes

I'll never forget my first pair of running shoes. I think I wore them for ten years! But times and technology have changed. Sport shoe manufacturers have invested a lot in researching and creating the right shoes for the right sport for the right people. There are running shoes for runners, tennis shoes for tennis players, and, in the late 80s, the aerobic and fitness worlds were blessed with special styles made just for them. Now, we can choose from walking shoes, aerobic shoes, step shoes, and cross-training shoes…so take the time to select from what's available and find the right shoe for your needs.

If you're an all-rounder, I'd suggest a cross-training shoe. This style allows you to participate comfortably in many different activities, from fitness training to traditional aerobic classes to walking outdoors.

If you prefer to specialize, and can invest the extra money, you will reap the benefits. A shoe specific to the type of training you do can make an enormous difference in performance. Also, with extra pairs of shoes, they'll all last longer. You should, at least, have a shoe just for outdoor sports activities and a separate pair for use indoors.

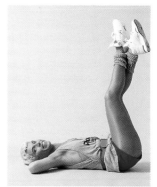

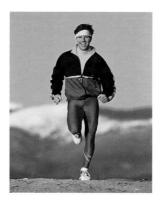

The clothing you wear during exercise should always be geared to the climactic conditions during training and to the type of exercise.

A hard workout—to burn fat, get in shape—and especially cardiovascular training is going to make you perspire. This cools the skin. So you don't

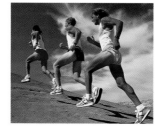

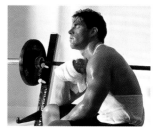

It's especially important when training outside, but don't forget to take the temperature in your indoor studio or training location into consideration.

get chilled, take precautions. Dress smart—in layers, like an onion! Having your own fitness equipment available is a great investment in your health.

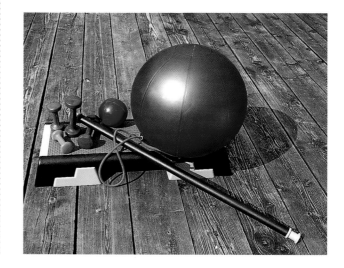

Equipped to Be Fit

Wearing a heart-rate monitor puts you in touch with your inner self! Then the watch you wear on your wrist not only keeps track of time, but measures your heart rate during training.

Step aerobics training was the first aerobic workout with muscle. It's an exercise for the whole-body that's as easy on the joints as walking, but is as cardio intense as running. A combination that can't be beat!

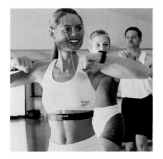

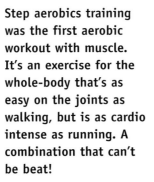

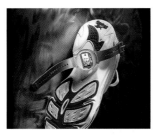

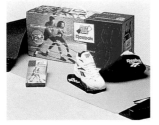

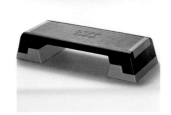

A "slide" device will help tone and define the thighs. It is great training for balance, and ice and in-line skating simulation. Just as important as clothing is your choice of shoes. Comfort and function have priority! When you cool down and stretch, you should be warm and dry.

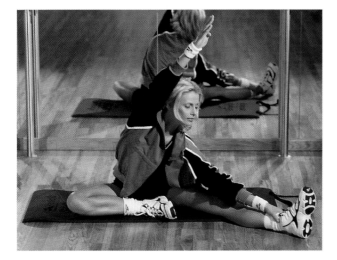

When you do shop, here is what to look for:

● *How is the cushioning?* You need good cushioning in the shoe to protect your joints. It should run through the mid-sole and, depending on the type of shoe, heavier under the forefoot (aerobic shoes) and the heel or both.

● *Do the shoes give you good medial and lateral support?* By this I mean, do the shoes prevent your feet from "tipping"—leaning to the inside, or outward. Support is found on the outer and inner edges of the shoe—the problem has nothing to do with the shoe's height. So, look for this medial and lateral support.

● *Does the shoe complement the form of your foot?* If you have a very broad forefoot, it is important to choose a shoe that will accommodate it. Nothing is worse than shoes that pinch. Your exercise performance will suffer for this bad choice.

● *Is the shoe long enough?* Your big toe should not push against the front of the shoe; nor should your foot slide back and forth in the shoe. Your heel should fit firmly in the shoe and stay in place.

● *Should you choose a low, mid, or high cut shoe?* It's entirely up to you; comfort is the main thing. High cuts may give you the feeling that your ankles are protected from tipping, but, as mentioned, that's a matter of lateral support, not shoe height.

Try on several pairs. Walk around, do sports moves, if space allows. Your feet are irreplaceable. Get a quality shoe that feels good; looks are secondary. Tip: Ask your podiatrist to prescribe special sport orthotics to replace the sock liner (removable in most brands) for a custom-made version of the same shoe!

Socks

Two words: Wear them! Buy pure cotton socks because they absorb sweat. Synthetics encourage athlete's foot and help create blisters. Wearing no socks is *not an option*! The shoe will suffer for it, your feet will suffer for it, and anyone near you will suffer, too, from the fumes emanating from well-worn sockless shoes!

Equipment and alternatives

A bodybar, hand weights, tubing, expander, rubber bands, platform, slide, training mat—all are very useful, if you use them! But, not ready for the investment or don't have the time to shop? Don't put off training until...whenever. Start now and use whatever is at hand: a pole or broom handle instead of a bodybar, a slice of bicycle inner tube or nylon stocking instead of tubing, a bicycle pump as an expander, bean-filled socks or bags as weights.

Keeping in touch

Two devices that will allow you to really become your own personal trainer are a digital blood-pressure monitor and a heart-rate monitor. These two pieces of monitoring equipment should be used each time you train in order to measure your internal progress and help you get in touch with your body.

III. Technique—Key to Moving Well

Your posture reveals more about you than any auto-biography ever will. Standing proud is not just an expression, it's a fact. If your shoulders are back and your chest is out, you look important and self-assured. If you make yourself stand tall even when you're not feeling well or good about yourself, you automatically open up and allow energy to flow in and out! If your poor posture is due to an injury or genetic factors, exercising properly will lead to great improvement.

Neutral Body Alignment—Good Posture

I grew up with classical ballet. The way I stood, every movement I made had to be perfect, from pointing my foot to the way I held my head. These principles have remained with me and have become my trademark in the fitness industry. Every one of my students, who go through the ranks of aerobic education with me, know that all their movements will be scrutinized. The aerobic department in our club is renowned for the good technique of not only my aerobic instructors but also our members, who are reminded of posture and correct execution of movement each time they come to class. So let's examine good posture. In fitness jargon, correct posture is called "the neutral position." I will continually refer to the neutral position for all the exercises in this book.

Your head should remain an extension of your spine. That means it is always to be held *upright;* you don't stick out your chin or lay it on your chest! Your shoulders are pressed down and back (it helps, here, to pinch your shoulder blades slightly together) and your chest is lifted. You have to consciously practice this at first. Now comes the hard part! The natural curve of the spine looks like the letter "S". The top of the "S" is the upper back, the swerve inward is the lower back, and the end of the "S" is our buttocks. Of course, our stance shouldn't be quite so exaggerated. If we learn to contract our abdominal muscles correctly—ribs to hip bones —which you will learn about in the exercise section on abdominals, you will train your muscles to hold your trunk so that you are automatically in a neutral position. Our trunk, or "core" as it is often called, is that part of our body that stabilizes us. If you have balance and coordination problems, strong trunk muscles will help improve these problems immensely. Don't confuse the neutral position with swayback, a postural problem which can also be helped through consistent muscle strength and stretching exercises.

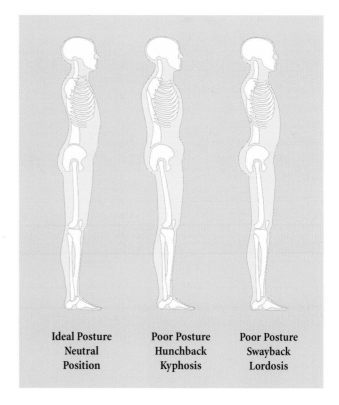

**Ideal Posture
Neutral
Position**

**Poor Posture
Hunchback
Kyphosis**

**Poor Posture
Swayback
Lordosis**

To find your neutral position, look at yourself sideways in a mirror. Stand straight, with knees slightly relaxed. Use your buttocks and stomach muscles to find your S-curve. If sway-backed, try to straighten the S-curve by pulling abdominal muscles together and slightly inwards. Distribute body weight evenly; not back (on heels) or forward (on balls of feet).

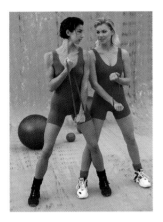

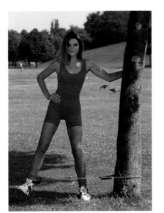

Neutral Wrist Position

Your wrist remains straight, as if a steel rod went from your hand to your elbow. Keeping this neutral position protects muscles and tendons in the wrist from strains when working with resistance equipment.

Neutral Foot Position

The neutral position shown here is a relaxed but stable foot. This means that you do not flex or point the foot. With this neutral position, all the energy stays in the working muscle.

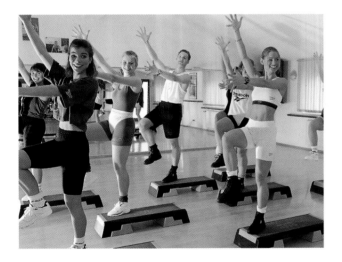

Neutral Body Position

Even while we move, we should maintain neutral posture: the head an extension of the spine, shoulders relaxed. These steppers, except the man in the middle, are demonstrating good posture!

Now that you've become aware of posture again (remember your mom saying "don't slouch"?—she was right!), try to practice standing, sitting and moving tall during all your daily activities

Something else that is important to think about: As we age, whether through osteoporosis or just the plain unvarnished fact of getting older, our spine starts to atrophy (shrink). If we fight against this process, with muscle training, stretching, and constant good posture, we'll look younger longer…and without the help of a plastic surgeon!

Most people suck in their stomach, tilt their pelvis and pinch their buttocks together, when told to stand correctly. Try doing this and then walk normally!

As I mentioned before, the best way to achieve good posture is to learn the rib-to-hip contraction. Here's how: Stand in a neutral position, place your thumb on your last rib (dig a little deeper, you'll find it) and the middle finger on your hip bone. Notice the distance between them. Now, still holding your fingers on the rib and hip bone, laugh—really laugh, "ha" "ha" "ha", breathing out hard with each "ha." If that doesn't work, try coughing deeply. Did you notice them move together? Now you have to learn to do this by simply contracting your abdominal muscles. You'll need a lot of concentration to do this at first. For some people it's not so easy and needs lots of practice. So keep on laughing!

Neutral Wrist Position

Most people's wrists are weak and therefore vulnerable to injury. They usually give way very quickly under pressure.

I will constantly remind you to maintain a neutral position of the wrist, while you are doing exercises that involve using hand weights, but especially with tubing and rubber bands. Let's take a bicep curl, for example. If you let the tubing pull your hand downwards, thus bending your wrist, you will be over-stretching the tendons, muscles and ligaments in your wrist. If you do this every time you exercise, you will strain your wrist joint—which would give you a good excuse to stop training!

Neutral Foot Position

I already explained that the neutral foot position is neither flexed nor pointed. This stable, relaxed foot position contributes to the so-called "specificity of training." If I am working my inner thigh muscles (see pages 107 and 108, exercises 19 and 20), I primarily want to contract the inner-thigh muscles—sounds logical, doesn't it? So why would I need to flex my foot, thus contracting the shin muscles, or point my foot, thus contracting my calf muscles? To efficiently train those two muscle groups, I have far better exercises.

I need the energy and concentration where I am working a specific muscle. A neutral foot helps the energy flow go where it's supposed to go!

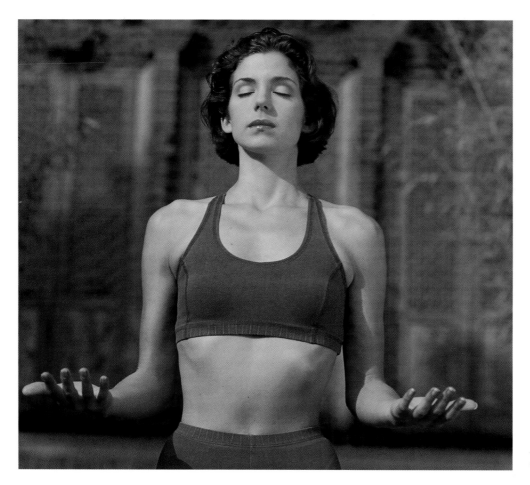

Deep breathing fills the body with energy.

Breathing Technique

For most of us, breathing is such a natural part of life that we really don't think about it until we get a cold or run out of it when we are exercising. The mechanics of breathing occur automatically through a rhythmic movement of your ribcage (thoracic cavity). When you breathe in, or inhale, your ribcage expands because the diaphragm, the muscle that forms the floor of the ribcage, contracts and rises; when you breathe out, or exhale, your ribcage sinks down and your diaphragm relaxes. When you inhale, blood is carried to the right side of the heart by way of the veins.

Breathing is both automatic and voluntary and is controlled by the nervous system, which is housed in a part of the spinal cord. This system continuously sends impulses to our respiratory muscles. Our breathing is affected by the amount of oxygen and the concentration of carbon monoxide in our blood. Breathing is also affected by our emotions.

I have learned that breathing is truly the connection between mind and body. With every conscious breath we take, we can literally fill our bodies up with energy. It is truly the key to mastering life's challenges and elevating mind and mood.

It's a sad fact that most people breathe just deeply enough to

Breathe In

Maria shows us how to do it right: You breathe in just before you begin the exercise, inhaling through the nose. Your mouth stays closed.

Do not inhale through the mouth. If you begin to hyperventilate or get dizzy, stop this exercise until you feel your breathing normalize.

Maria does it right: When we contract our muscles during an exercise, we breathe out through our mouths.

keep from falling over unconscious! Neuroscientists report that we are not supplying our brains with optimal levels of oxygen.

Another sad surprise, according to a five-year study done by Dr. James J. Lynch of the Center for the Study of Human Psychophysiology at the University of Maryland School of Medicine, is that poor breathing contributes to high blood pressure. If you don't take in enough oxygen through breathing, your blood has to circulate more rapidly to compensate and carry the same amount of oxygen. This can result in an increase in blood pressure, because our blood has to move faster to maintain the oxygen supply.

Proper breathing technique is of primary importance when we exercise. Oxygen helps to produce ATP (adenosine triphosphate), a chemical energy molecule needed in virtually all cells of the body. Without sufficient ATP, we cannot contract our muscles, or even think clearly!

The goal of good breathing technique is to take in a lot of oxygen with each breath. Naturally, it is important to consider the quality of the oxygen taken in. Make sure that when you exercise you have access to fresh air. Remember that cardiovascular exercise is designed to enhance oxygen intake. Practice inhaling and exhaling deeply. Try to exhale longer than you inhale. This way you expel toxins from the crevices of your lungs. I think of it as emptying the garbage.

Very important for all the exercises: Breathe in through the nose, and out through the mouth!

Breathing from the diaphragm

Diaphragmatic breathing, as it is called, is a far more efficient breathing technique in comparison to chest breathing. First of all, it utilizes far less energy to bring in far more oxygen to your body. It also expels the used oxygen far more efficiently.

Let's practice breathing through the diaphragm: Lay down on your back. Put your right hand just under your chest and your left hand on your stomach. Breathe in. Which hand came up higher? Now concentrate and purposely push your stomach out when you breathe in. Now when you breathe out flatten it, pushing your back into the floor.

Tip: Place your hands lightly around the sides of your lower ribs with the fingertips pointing in toward the navel. Your thumbs are to the rear. Slowly inhale through the nose. Feel how the abdomen expands and how the ribs move out to the sides. Touching the outside of the lower ribs gives a signal to the brain which improve your results.

Chest breathing

This is a common, but far more inefficient, method of breathing. Only the chest wall muscles, rather than the diaphragm, act to take in oxygen, so only the top and mid-part of the lungs are filled, not the lower part, which is where most blood techanges take place. Also less carbon monoxide is expelled. Because the dia-phragm is not being fed with sufficient oxygen, we often suffer from side stitches during sport. If you've been working out very hard cardiovascularly, and are breathing very heavily, you will automatically be doing chest breathing. You won't have the time or energy enough to practice diaphragmatic breathing.

Deep breathing

Breathing deeply is not only beneficial to exercise, but a wonderful way to rid your body of stress. Whenever you are tense, angry, or generally out of control, practice this little two-step exercise:

Exhale completely—really blow out all the air in your lungs, so that your ribs and stomach are totally flat. First step: breathe in using the diaphragmatic technique—your stomach should be distended. Second step: in the same breath fill your lungs and extend your ribcage. Now, when you exhale, reverse the process: first breathe out, letting the air out of the lungs and then out of the diaphragm. It's kind of like a wave!

Remember that for all the exercises in this book you will inhale *before* beginning the exercise, exhale *during* the exercise or contraction and then inhale *as* you relax or release. The only exceptions to this rule are exercises for the lower back and the muscles that run along the spine. With these exercises, you should find your own rhythm and breathe naturally.

Body Alignment and Placement

I have already introduced you to postural alignment, with the neutral position. When we stand our shoulders should be over the hips, the hips and knees over the middle of our feet. Every position and every movement has its own alignment. When you do a lunge, for example, your front leg is in a 90-degree angle, the alignment for the knee is over the heel of the foot, your shoulders are over the middle of your thigh and your back leg is extended behind you. Your body is in a diagonal line. This is the alignment for that movement.

Placement is where the distribution of weight should be. If we take the lunge again, three quarters our weight is placed over the front leg. If you do a jumping jack, you land on both feet with the weight evenly distributed onto both feet. With a static squat the weight would lie more in the heels.

Range of Motion

When you move a limb, or do an exercise, it is important that the muscles are used to their full extent. We call that using the full range of motion. For example, if you do an overhead press, you want to extend your arms completely out over your head.

Stretching is the best time to notice how little range of motion we have. If you cannot even clasp your hands together behind your back, the range of motion in your shoulder joint is extremely

Alignment and Placement

Example 1
Daniela is standing in a lunge position for calf exercises (see ex. 1, p. 113).

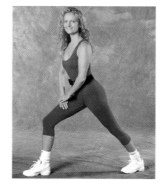

Example 2
Loren is doing door squats to exercise her buttocks muscles (see ex. 5, p. 94)

Alignment:
● **Shoulders are over the thighs, and her body builds a diagonal line from head to heels.**
● **Her front knee is in position directly over her heel.**

Placement:
● **Daniela's weight is three quarters over the front leg.**

● **Tips: To protect joints, stay within the correct range of motion, don't overextend. If you tend to "hyperextend," stop short of full extension and tense working muscle. Perform all movements**

Alignment:
● **Knees are slightly behind the heels and shoulders over thighs.**
● **Knees and feet are slightly turned out; feet flat and knees in line with foot direction.**
● **Arms are at shoulder height, almost extended.**

Placement:
● **Weight is on her heels.**

slowly, with control and concentration.
When you jump, roll down the toe, ball, and heel, and bend your knees. This cushions the impact, protecting the joints and spine.

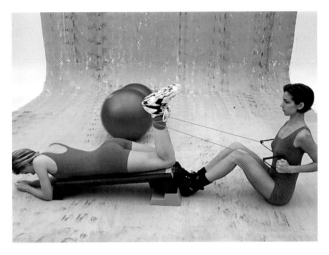

Wrapping

What is wrapping? How do I "wrap" a foot or leg? How do I attach a wrap to a tree or other object?

tubing ends are even. To wrap a tree, pole or other convenient object, lay the tubing around it (it must be something

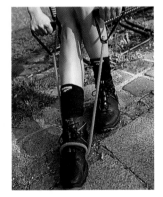

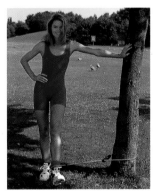

For a footwrap, lay the tubing over the top and wind both ends around the bottom of the foot. Make sure ends are even. For a legwrap, lay the tubing just above the ankle at the front of the leg. Wind it around to the back, making sure

stable, that doesn't move). Pull one end of the tubing through the other, forming a loop or "handle." Now, pull a piece of the tubing through the handle to form a foot loop, and you have a handy cable pulley. Clever, isn't it?

limited. There are. however, some people who should be very careful with use of range of motion. A person who has a chronic problem with shoulder dislocation should strengthen the rotator cuff muscles but avoid extreme stretches or movements that externally rotate the arm when it is in a raised position.

Please pay attention to the guidelines I have set for each exercise, and don't forget to read the tips. In this way, you will truly reap benefits from your training.

Hyperextension and Hyperflexion

Good technique means not overextending joints or the spine. A hyperextension of the arm looks as if you are bending it *backwards*. Some people call this being double-jointed. This is especially common in women. What it really means, however, is that the muscles haven't put on the brakes, stopping the overextension, and that the ligaments of that joint are probably lax. People who can carry out unnatural stretches, going beyond their normal range of motion, often develop massive problems with their joints later in life. Osteoarthritis and degenerative joint problems are very common among ex-ballet dancers and former gymnasts. As non-professionals, you don't have to expose your body to these extremes.

A word to pregnant women: Your bodies produce a hormone during pregnancy that relaxes the muscles, tendons, and ligaments around the joints. Hyperextension and hyperflexion are a real danger, so stay in your normal range of motion. If you are double-jointed, muscle strength exercises are an absolute must!

Tubes, Bands, and the Various "Wraps"

I love working with tubing (or "tubes" as they're often called) and rubber bands. They are light and easily transportable, so you really have no excuse to leave them behind when you travel.

When attaching the tubing to objects, make sure that the looped tubing is really in place and correct…and that the object is not going to move! I once attached tubing to the leg of a cupboard and almost pulled the cupboard over onto myself as I was doing my exercise! Also, every time that you go to use your tubing and rubber bands, check them over for signs of weakness and wear and tear.

Tubing and rubber bands come in different strengths. If you plan to progress in your training, as you should, it might be a good idea now to invest in three different strengths! Actually, you may even need to use a stronger tube in exercising one body-part and a weaker one for another!

IV. The Exercises

Did you know that your body is made up of more than 650 muscles that you can move voluntarily? And did you know that there are even more muscles that move involuntarily?

Our bodies contain three types of muscle tissue: skeletal muscle (biceps, triceps, quadriceps, etc.), smooth muscle (in the walls of the arteries and the gastrointestinal tract), and cardiac muscle (the heart).

The skeletal muscles are the muscles over which we normally have control; they are voluntary. When we are doing an exercise, we tell our brain to send a message to the muscles, and the muscle fibers react by contracting—getting shorter. Just like conscious breathing, muscle training is a mind-body connection.

The skeletal muscles are attached to the bones by tendons. Ligaments connect bones to other bones at a joint. The skeletal muscles produce the strength for the movement we wish to make. The tendons transmit this muscle strength to the bones, allowing the joints to move in the desired way.

Every joint is surrounded by a group of muscles that help to stabilize and to move it.

It is quite a complex system of transmission that controls movements in the human body.

Muscle Function

There are many things to consider with muscle function. The simplest and most understandable is the principle of positive and negative, push and pull—that one muscle is the primary mover (the agonist), responsible for producing the movement, and the other (the antagonist) opposes the primary mover, demonstrates the properties of extensibility. A muscle can be an agonist one time and the next time it might play the role of antagonist. If you bend your lower arm up to your shoulder, your bicep is the agonist and your tricep is playing the part of the antagonist. Now, if you stretch your arm out again, your tricep is the agonist and the bicep is the antagonist! In addition to these two muscles, many other muscles come into play, assisting and stabilizing, in order to complete the called-for movement.

Although the antagonist is called the opposing muscle, when it produces tension, i.e., when the muscle contracts eccentrically, it is actually serving as a brake system, controlling the movement of the agonist.

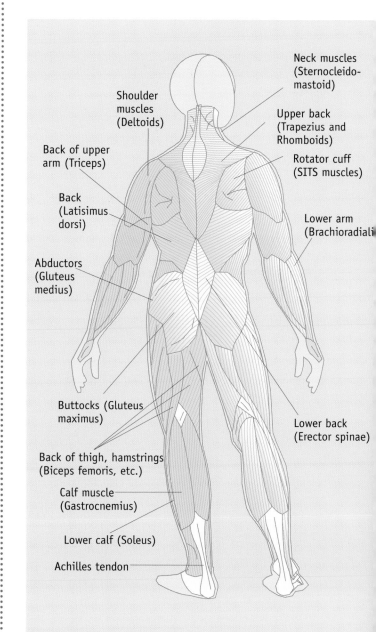

Shoulder muscles (Deltoids)

Neck muscles (Sternocleido-mastoid)

Upper back (Trapezius and Rhomboids)

Back of upper arm (Triceps)

Rotator cuff (SITS muscles)

Back (Latisimus dorsi)

Lower arm (Brachioradiali

Abductors (Gluteus medius)

Buttocks (Gluteus maximus)

Lower back (Erector spinae)

Back of thigh, hamstrings (Biceps femoris, etc.)

Calf muscle (Gastrocnemius)

Lower calf (Soleus)

Achilles tendon

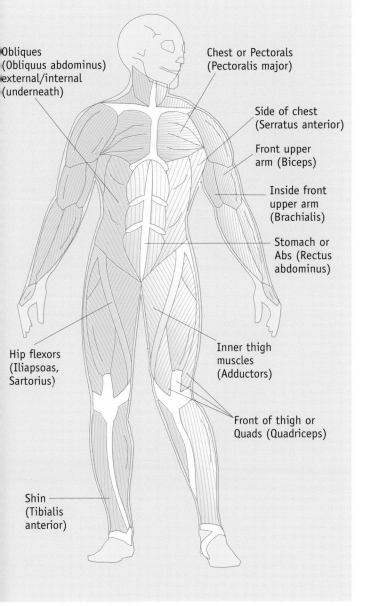

Obliques (Obliquus abdominus) external/internal (underneath)

Chest or Pectorals (Pectoralis major)

Side of chest (Serratus anterior)

Front upper arm (Biceps)

Inside front upper arm (Brachialis)

Stomach or Abs (Rectus abdominus)

Hip flexors (Iliapsoas, Sartorius)

Inner thigh muscles (Adductors)

Front of thigh or Quads (Quadriceps)

Shin (Tibialis anterior)

The Main Muscles

There are various skeletal muscles, which produce different movements or actions and are found in different parts of the body:

The trunk and hip muscles include the stomach muscles, the lower back, the hip flexors, and the buttocks.

The muscles of the upper extremities include the chest, upper back, and the shoulders and arm muscles.

The muscles of the lower extremities include the legs and calves, and again the buttocks (which connect trunk and legs).

Goal-Oriented Muscle Training

For those of you who wish to really make positive and *realistic* changes in your body, you have to give a lot of thought to mapping out your exercise plan. It is essential to acquaint yourself with the main muscle groups or body parts, which will be introduced in the following exercises. Naturally, you will not only be training those targeted muscles but many other muscles that have not been named here.

At the beginning of each exercise chapter, we will introduce you to the muscle that you will be exercising, and explain its characteristics, plus any specific information that will help you to understand its mechanics.

Shoulders

Release

the Tension

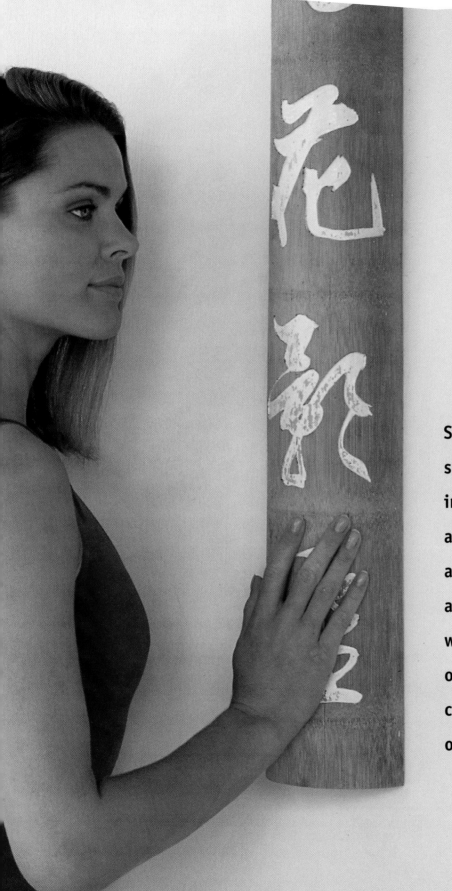

Strong, attractive
shoulders not only
influence your whole
appearance: relaxed
and tension-free neck
and shoulder muscles
will release you from
one of the most
common maladies of
our time—headaches!

Exercises for the Shoulders

Shoulders define our stature. They influence our appearance far more than any other body part. Broad, well defined but relaxed shoulders are a sign of strength and self-confidence.

Just as broad, beautiful shoulders contribute to your appearance, tense, tight shoulder muscles, on the other hand, will cause discomfort and pain. Because of this, it is very important to train this body part with equal doses of strengthening and stretching exercises.

If you suffer from tension headaches and feel (and look like) your shoulders are stuck to your ears, then your first priority will be to stretch the shoulder area.

In my first session with my clients, I always give them "homework"—and this is your first session with me, so pay attention. Try to notice every time your shoulders are tensed up.

Pull them down and hold them down. Do this throughout your day. You'll really be so surprised at how often you automatically tense your shoulders up. The shoulder is a ball and socket joint. It is the most mobile joint in the body and therefore one of the most in danger of injury, especially dislocation. Because of this, it is important to secure its strength through specific exercises.

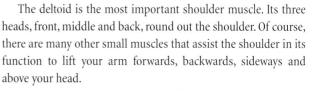

The deltoid is the most important shoulder muscle. Its three heads, front, middle and back, round out the shoulder. Of course, there are many other small muscles that assist the shoulder in its function to lift your arm forwards, backwards, sideways and above your head.

Some of the shoulder exercises will run over only one joint. For example, exercise 1, shoulder raises. You will lift your arm, holding it in a straight line, thus not changing the angle of the movement. The whole arm is literally lifted by the front shoulder muscle. This means that the elbow and the wrist stay straight for the entire exercise.

You'll also perform a two-joint exercise. The upright row with tubing, exercise 7, is an example of movement in two joints. You will bend your elbows and lift with your shoulders, your wrist will be held straight. Remember to perform all exercises in a slow and controlled manner.

Guidelines for Exercising the Shoulders

❶ **Do not work with momentum; that means, don't *swing* your arms up. *Bring* them up with your muscles. Also, don't swing your body in order to achieve the movement. Stand firm!**

❷ **Keep your shoulders down. Your head remains a continuation of your spine, i.e., it doesn't move while you are doing the exercise.**

❸ **Pay attention to how the hands are held during the exercise. If you turn the hands outward or inward by certain exercises, you change the way the shoulder works. This can cause impingement, especially when the arms are brought overhead. So pay attention to the hands!**

❹ **When you contract, breathe out; when you release or relax, breathe in.**

1. Shoulder Raise Combo with Hand Weights

Starting Position

Sit on a chair where you arms can move freely; back straight, feet flat on the floor. Begin with arms slightly bent but tensed, held next to your hips. Wrists are neutral. Maria is holding two one-pound weights. Choose the weight suited to your level. This is a muscle endurance exercise, so you will be doing more reps.

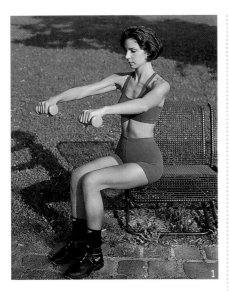

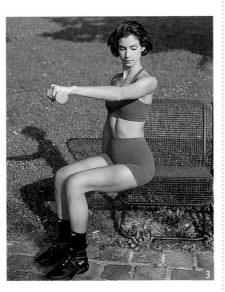

Step 1

Slowly lift both of your arms straight up to shoulder level. Slowly lower them. Now, raise just your right arm slowly, and then lower it. Concentrate, and control your movements.

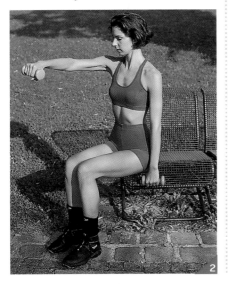

Step 2

Bring both arms up again and lower them. Now raise your left arm and lower it. Now repeat the whole combination: both arms, right arm, both arms, left arm.

Reps

 No combo, just arms 8–16×
Whole sequence 8–16×

Tip

Don't throw your arms up; lift them slowly, keeping the arms tense. Lift them only to shoulder height.
This exercise trains the front shoulder muscles.

2. Overhead Press with Bodybar

Starting Position

Amanda shows start position. Hold bar (stick or pole) with palms down. Arms are chest height, feet shoulder-width apart with knees slightly bent.

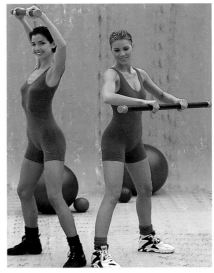

Exercise

Raise bar upwards, stopping in line with your forehead (not directly over your head). Maria's arms remain slightly bent but tensed. Slowly lower the arms. This exercise trains the middle shoulder muscle.

Reps

With pole 8–20×
With bodybar 8–20×
(or 3 sets of 8)

Tip

For more range of motion, start with the bodybar down near your thighs. Don't use your body to *throw* the weight up. Stand firm and raise the bar with your shoulder muscles.

3. Overhead Press with Tubing

4. Double-Duty Bicep Pull-Ups (partner does back rows)

Starting Position

Sit with a straight back on a bench or in a chair, leaning slightly forward from the hips. Pass the tubing under a bench or chair. Hold the tubing handles securely at shoulder height, with the knuckles towards the ceiling. *Make sure that your wrists are in neutral position!*

Starting Position

Stand with feet apart, knees flexed. Hold tubing, elbow at 90 degrees. Partner kneels, leg out. Holds tubing with arms tucked, shoulders down.

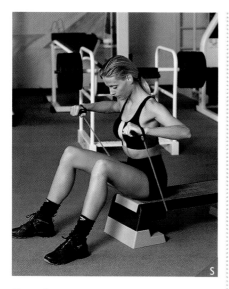
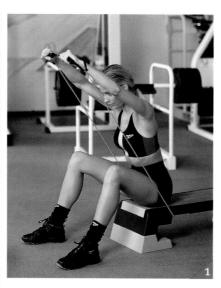
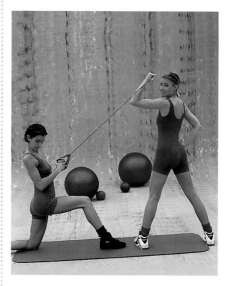

Exercise

Extend the arms slightly forward and upwards. Don't stretch out the arms completely. Breathe out when bringing the arms upwards. Breathe in when you lower them.

Variation

You can also perform this exercise with hand weights or free weights. If you choose this type of resistance, make sure the weight allows for good technique.

Reps

 Light tubing or weights 8–12×
Middle to heavy tubing or weights 8–20×, or 3× 8 sets

Exercise

Doing back rows, Maria pulls on tubing with both hands, keeping arms close to her sides. Amanda pulls the tubing upward toward the ceiling; the arm remains steady in the 90-degree angle. Kneeling partner changes leg at arm change.

Reps

 8–12×; change arms
8–20×; change arms

Info

If you really concentrate and lower the tubing slowly you can feel the muscles in the back working. A plus of this exercise is that the tricep muscle is also worked.

Tip

Though you lean slightly forward, your back remains straight. You control the tubing; the tubing does not control you. Especially on the way down! This exercise trains the middle shoulder muscles.

Tip

Remember, work your arms, not your body, to complete the pull-ups. The wrist always remains neutral! Amanda's exercise, the pull-ups, trains the front and middle shoulder muscles.

5. Bicep Pull-Ups with Tubing

Starting Position
Stand with one foot forward, knees flexed, feet pointing forward, tubing fixed firmly under front foot. Center weight between feet. See Debbie's left arm position for the start position of the arms; that is, at a 90-degree angle and held close to the body. The elbows are back, and backs of hands towards the floor.

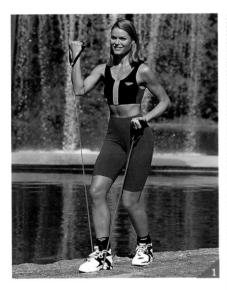 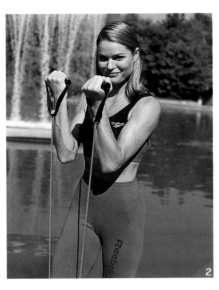

Step 1
Keeping the arm in the 90-degree angle, raise the right arm so that the elbow is level with your shoulder. Keep your shoulders down and your wrists neutral. Slowly bring the arm down to the start position. Both raising and lowering are to be performed in a slow and controlled manner.

Step 2
Now perform the above movements with both arms. Watch your wrists; your knuckles point to the ceiling.

Step 3
Now do Step 1 with the left arm.

Step 4
To finish, repeat the Step 2 combo: right arm up and down, then both arms, then left, then both again.

Reps
- Whole combo 4–8×, or each combo as a set, 4–8 sets
- Whole combo 8–16×

Tip

For beginners, it is better to rest between each combo and make sets out of them.
Be careful not to lean backwards when lifting the arms up. This is hard to do, so practice each movement individually before doing the combo.
This exercise trains the front and middle shoulder muscles.

6. Side Lateral Raises with Tubing

Starting Position
Take Debbie's position in exercise 5. Hold your arms like Amanda is doing, at your sides and slightly bent. The shoulders are down, wrists are neutral.

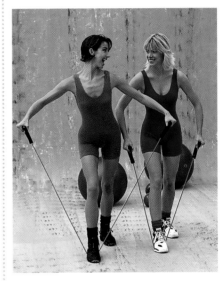

Exercise
Pull your arms upward to the sides, with the elbows leading the movement. Palms face down. Don't pull up any higher than shoulder level and don't drop your elbows down.

Reps
- 8–16×
- With tubing under both feet 8–16×

Tip

Stand steady, don't lean back. Don't drop your elbows or pull the tubing higher than shoulder level. And *keep your wrists neutral!* This exercise trains the middle shoulder muscles.

7. Upright Row with Tubing

Starting Position
As in exercise 5. Lay tubing handles together and hold with both hands. See arm and hand positions below. Keep a neutral body alignment.

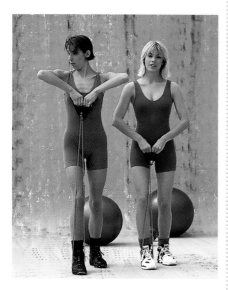

Exercise
Pull the tubing up, keeping your elbows out and your shoulders down. Lower it down slowly to the starting position.

Reps
⊏▭⊐ 8–12×
⊟▭⊟ 8–20×

Tip
When pulling the tubing up, try to lead with your elbows. Keep a neutral position and don't lean or fall back as you pull up on the tubing. Watch your wrists—keep a neutral wrist at all times! This exercise trains the middle shoulder muscles.

8. Bow and Arrow with Rubber Bands

Starting Position
As Amanda is demonstrating, stand in a modified lunge. Both feet should be pointing forward, both front leg and back leg slightly bent. Hold the rubber band as if it were a bow and arrow. One arm is extended; the other is bent at shoulder height. The palms of your hands face towards the floor.

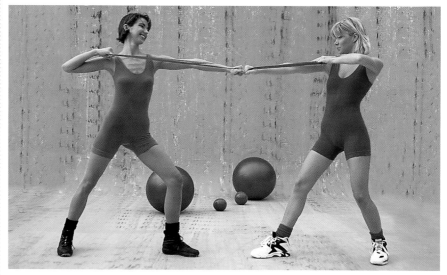

Exercise
Bring your bent arm back, as if you were pulling on a bow. You should feel your shoulder blade move towards the middle of your back. Keep the elbow at shoulder height throughout the exercise. Slowly bring the pulling arm back to the starting position. Maintain tension in the band at all times.

Reps
⊏▭⊐ 8–12×
⊟▭⊟ 8–20×

Important
Keep your abdominal muscles pulled together and in. In the lunge position, watch your alignment. Knee over heel, shoulders over the hips, head straight. Don't forget your breathing techniques.

Tip
If you are more advanced, take a deeper lunge, like Maria's: front leg bent, back leg a little more extended. Your trunk, chest, and back stay steady during the exercise. Keep the palms facing the floor as you pull back, don't twist the arm. Keep wrists neutral. This exercise trains the rear shoulder muscles. (It also trains the rhomboids, which lie under the trapezius.)

9. Pull-Backs with Tubing

Starting Positions
This is one of my favorite exercises. Sit very straight in a chair that allows you to move your arms straight back. Your arms are fully extended, your abdominals pulled in, shoulders down. Now, try to pull your shoulder blades just a little bit together. Your knuckles face the floor and wrists remain in neutral position (this is very important). Use the footwrap around one foot (see page 35).

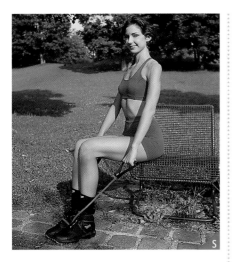
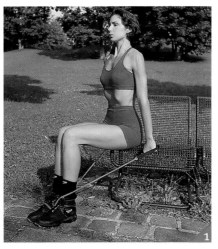

Exercise
Tighten the stomach and raise the chest slightly. Now, pull the tubing back, keeping the arms and wrists absolutely straight! Try to hold it in position for the count of 2, then slowly bring the arms back to start. Take a deep breath before you start again, and really exhale with power when you pull back.

Reps
8–12×
8–12×, 3 sets

Tip
It is very important to keep the wrists straight. If you bend them, they not only risk being strained but the effect of the exercise is reduced.

Tip
Keep your trunk very straight. For more tension, either use heavier tubing, or put the footwrap around both feet (over the top of the feet, wind around the back of the feet, bring both tubing ends between the feet, and hold them on the side of the legs). This exercise trains the rear shoulder muscles and statically trains the trunk, especially the abdominal muscles.

10. Rear Shoulder Stretches

Starting Position
Stand in a neutral position, feet shoulder width apart. Clasp your hands behind your back, keep the arms extended and pull them downwards.

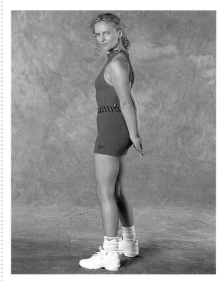

Really push the shoulders downwards as you pull the arms down further. You can also raise the arms up slightly to feel even more pull in the front of your shoulder muscles. Hold: 20–30 seconds, shake out the arms and repeat.

Tip
If you want to stretch your neck muscles as well, drop your chin to your chest and hold the position 20–30 seconds. Remember to inhale and exhale deeply during the stretch.

Chest

Make the Best

of Your Chest!

A word to the women: Strong chest muscles will not make you into a 36C, but they will give you more definition and support for the fatty tissues that make up the breasts.

As for you men: well, a broad chest *is* the very best!

Exercises for the Chest

In order to accomplish certain tasks in our daily life, we use our upper bodies in many different positions. We use our arms to push and pull in front, downwards, and over our heads. In order to accomplish these movements, our chest muscles should be exercised at various angles in order to meet the demands of their function.

There is something all of us should know by now: The size of the female breast is something that is either genetically determined or "remedied" at the plastic surgeon's. Exercising the muscles of the chest will *not* enlarge the breasts.

The breasts are made up of fatty tissue; if you gain weight, you also usually gain a little more in breast size. Exercising the pectoral muscles, as they are called, will help with posture and give you definition and stature. It will also aid in strengthening the arms for various movements. Due to our daily routines, the pectorals are one of the tightest and shortened muscles. This causes our shoulders to curve inwards. If you look in the mirror and see this posture staring back at you, please stretch your pectorals for a week or two before starting the prescribed chest exercises.

You have two main chest muscles, the pectoral major and minor. Put your right hand over the front of the left side of your chest and armpit. Now, raise the left arm and pull it inwards as if against an immovable object. You should feel the pectoralis contract. If you are a well-developed male, you can see the bulge that forms your pectoralis. (The pectorals in women are only visible in the upper part of the chest and the armpit, because they are covered with breasts in the lower part.) This muscle contributes immensely to rotation in the shoulder girdle. The pectoralis minor lies too deep to be seen.

All the exercises in this chapter should be carried out slowly and with control. Technique is of utmost importance. Therefore, it's appropriate here to introduce you to a correct push-up.

Push-ups are a great all-round exercise for the upper body. They train the shoulder girdle, but mainly really get to those pectoral and tricep muscles. Push-ups are an essential exercise! I know, ladies, that you hate this exercise. But give me a chance to prove to you that you, too, can do them well, even if you've never done them before or if you have tried and failed.

Technique Tips for Push-Ups

❶ **Take care not to overestimate your strength. If the exercise you are doing is too hard for you, go a level lower until you have the correct technique down.**
❷ **Whatever level you chose, remember to pull your abdominals together. Pinch your gluteals (bottom) tight and imagine that, from your head to the end of your bottom, you are a straight board. If you let your stomach sag in the middle you will be stressing your back.**
❸ **Inhale before you start the exercise and exhale as you push up. While you are in the up position, breathe in again.**
❹ **Start doing the exercise from the down position, with bent arms.**

48

1. Praying Press Standing

Starting Position

Stand in neutral position with feet placed shoulder-width apart and toes pointed forward. Place your forearms and hands together, with your fingertips pointed towards the ceiling. Pull your shoulders down and relax your neck muscles.

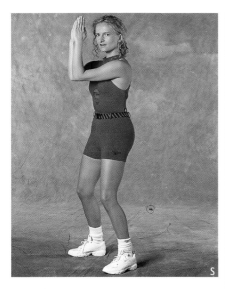

Exercise

Press your hands together and hold for 8–10 seconds. Relax. Now bring your forearms together, press again and hold for 8–10 seconds.

Reps

2–4×
4–8×

Info

This exercise is isometric. This means that the muscle we are exercising doesn't change in length but is tensed.
Your own arms and hands are the resistance, and are helping produce tension, or an isometric contraction, in the upper-chest muscles.

Tip

Press the shoulders down during the entire exercise.
If you want to work your glutes and abs (bottom and stomach) tilt your pelvis forward and pinch your buttocks together.

2. Chest Press with Baby

Starting Position

Lay prone, with feet flat and legs bent, holding your baby up like Daniela is holding Valentina here. Arms are bent, with elbows outwards.

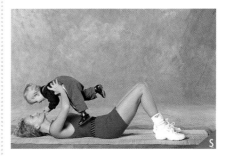

Exercise

Now to start. Daniela presses Valentina straight up in front of her chest, and then lowers her slowly back to start.

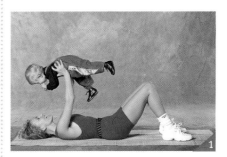

Reps

4–8×, up to 3 sets
8–12×, 3 sets

Tip

If you're not a young mother, use a bodybar or hand weights. When pushing up with the arms, be careful not to hyperextend the elbows.

3. Butterflies in Sitting Position with Partner

4. Chest Press Combo with Bodybar on a Platform

Starting Position
Your partner serves as a machine that works chest, shoulder, and arm muscles both positively and negatively (agonist and antagonist). Sit in a chair with partner behind. Hold arms shoulder height at 90-degree angle, back straight, shoulders pressed down, stomach contracted. The partner grasps your forearms.

Starting Position
Lay on a bench or step, your legs bent and feet flat on floor. Hold the bodybar at chest level. Keep upper arm and elbow in line with shoulder.

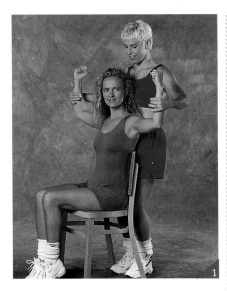
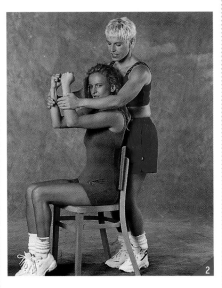

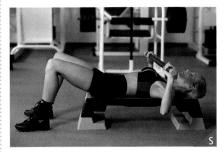

Exercise
Push arms slowly up towards the ceiling. Watch the elbows. Extend the arms, but be careful not to hyperextend them. Slowly lower the bodybar to the start position.

Step 1
Pull your arms slowly but fluidly inwards. Your partner applies resistance by pressing lightly on the inside of your forearms. Keep your shoulders down and back straight. Rest your head lightly against your partner and don't move it. If your partner increases the pressure so that you cannot move your arms anymore, the exercise becomes static or isometric.

Communicate with one another: If you are doing the exercise, you should direct your partner to apply the right dose of resistance. Your partner, acting here as your "trainer," has to adjust the application of resistance to your needs.

Step 2
When your arms are closed, your partner moves his/her hands to the outside of your forearms. As you push your arms open, your partner applies pressure. In this way, you are training the back muscles (the antagonist to the chest muscles). You can have your partner apply more pressure to make this exercise also static or isometric.

Reps
🔗 8–12×, 2× static, hold 10 seconds
🔗 8–16×, 4× static, hold 10 seconds

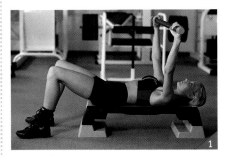

Reps
🔗 8–24×, weight up to 10 lbs.
🔗 8–12×, choose weight with rep limit under 12

Tip
Don't turn this exercise into a tug-of-war. This exercise is about getting a feeling for resistance and strength.

Tip
Alternative: free or hand weights. If you don't have a step or bench, do this exercise on the floor. Using a step or bench gives you more range of motion.

5. Chess Press Combo with Hand Weights on a Platform

Starting Position
Loren is lying in a supine position on a flat step. Her legs are hip-width apart. Instead of a bodybar, she is holding free weights. Her wrists are in a neutral position and will remain so throughout the exercise. Her arms are in a 90 degree angle with elbows in line with her shoulders. Loren inhales.

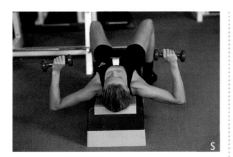

Step 1
Loren pushes the weights upwards and begins to exhale.

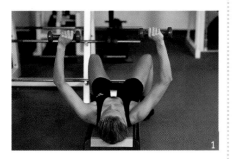

Step 2
Loren rotates her arms and hands inwards so that her palms are facing one another. As her arms and the hand weights come together, keeping her elbows slightly bent, she continues to exhale.

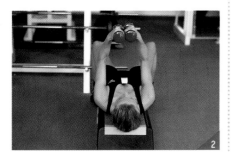

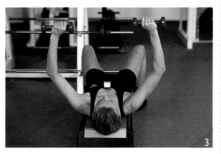

Step 3
Opening her arms to the position in Step 1, she begins to inhale.

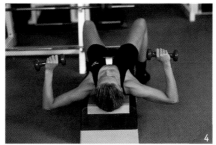

Step 4
Loren lowers her arms to the starting position and continues to inhale.

Reps
- With light weights 8–16×
- With heavier weights 8–12×

Tip
Keep the movements slow and fluid. Breathe out on the first two movements and in on the last two.

6. Double-Duty Chest and Abs Exercise on an Inclined Platform

Starting Position
Lie with head and shoulders slightly raised, legs shoulder-width apart. Upper arms, at 90-degree angle, align with shoulders. Palms face forward.

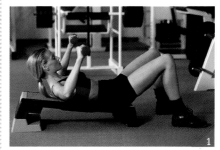

Step 1
In the above position, your chin a fist length from your sternum, inhale and start to squeeze your abs together. Remember to keep your buttocks relaxed.

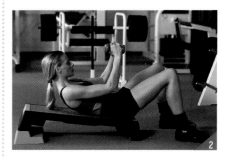

Step 2
Rotate arms inwards, so your palms are facing. Really exhale on this movement and pull abs in and even more tightly together, then contract chest muscles. Bottoms of shoulder blades remain on platform. Slowly roll back to start. Keep head and shoulders immobile throughout exercise.

Reps
- Advanced only: 8–12×, do slowly with lots of concentration

7. Supine Chest Pullover on an Inclined Platform

Starting Position
Loren here holds two 4 lb. weights. Her arms are bent. forearms facing the ceiling, palms facing one another. Her legs are hip width, feet flat on floor.

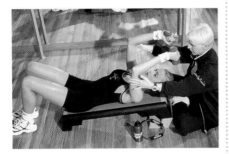

Exercise
Keeping her arms parallel to one another and in a 90-degree angle (I'm helping her here!), Loren pulls her elbows towards her chest, consciously squeezing her chest muscles together and exhaling. Slowly she returns her arms to the starting position.

Reps
⬤ With light weights 8-16×
⬤ With heavier weights 8-12×

8. Supine Chest Flye

Starting Position
Loren lies on a flat step. Her feet, shoulder-width apart, are firmly on the floor. Her head and shoulder blades are pressed tightly against the bench. Her arms rise straight up from her shoulders, weights held directly in line with her nose. Her elbows are flexed and rotated outwards, palms facing inwards. She inhales.

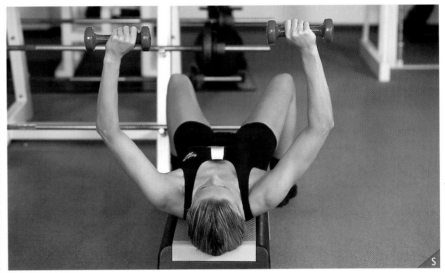

Exercise
Loren pulls her shoulder blades together tightly and tries to maintain the contraction throughout the entire exercise. Exhaling, she slowly lowers her arms to shoulder level, keeping her elbows slightly flexed. She inhales. Then, exhaling, she contracts her chest muscles and brings her arms slowly back up to the starting position.

Reps
⬤ With light weights 4–8×
⬤ With heavier weights 8–12×

Tip
This exercise can also be done holding one weight with both hands. To make this exercise even more advanced, turn around and do it in a decline position

Info
This exercise works the chest in adduction and abduction. This means that the tension in the muscles occurs when the muscles are shortened (arms going up) and lengthened (arms going down).

Tip
When bringing the arms upwards, visualize squeezing a big beach ball between your arms. Avoid any rotation in your elbows or wrists.

9. Push-Ups on the Floor

Level 1

Loren and I show you the starting position for beginners (a mat or towel under the knees is a kindness). Start on all fours, forehead touching the floor, arms bent an upper-arm length from your shoulders. Fingers should either point forward or be just slightly turned out. The trunk is held straight as a board—your ab muscles pulled together so your back doesn't collapse. The lower legs stay on the floor throughout the exercise. Now slowly extend your arms, lifting your body.

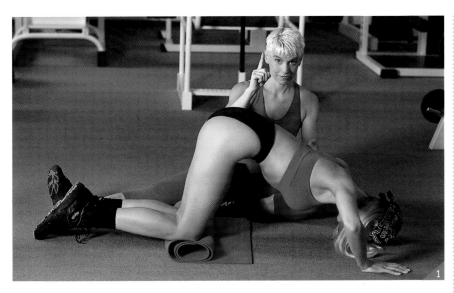

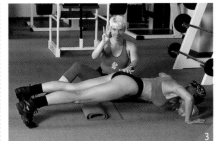

Level 3

Loren does all the work, while I simply indicate the levels. In these advanced "pro push-ups," start on the floor with arms as above, legs extended, feet flexed to work from the balls of the feet. Again, keeping the whole body straight as a board, extend the arms and lift your body from the floor as one unit. Lower yourself; but not completely to the floor; start again from that point. Keep buttocks and ab muscles tensed at all times.

Level 2

Start by lying face down on the floor, arm position as in level 1. Lift your lower legs and keep them up during the entire exercise. Slowly push your head, trunk, and thighs simultaneously away from the floor by extending your arms. Make very sure that the body, from head to knee, is kept absolutely straight—as if it were a board! Don't let your back collapse into your stomach, creating a swayback.

Reps

- Level 1: slowly 8–12×;
- Level 2: slowly 8–12×;
- Level 3 (pro): set 1 slowly 8–16×; set 2 a bit faster 8–16× (if able); set 3 slowly!

Tip

Push-ups save time because you train chest and triceps together. Remember, it's better to do fewer repetitions correctly, using proper technique. This way the muscles really get a workout.

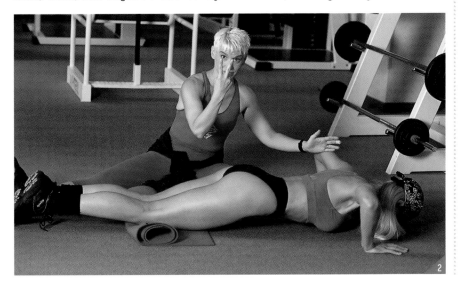

10. Push-Ups on the Wall

Starting Position
Daniela's body position is just like Loren's in Step 3 of exercise 9, except that she is in a standing position. She stands far enough from the wall so that she can extend her arms almost completely when she pushes herself away from the wall. Notice that her hands are turned slightly inwards.

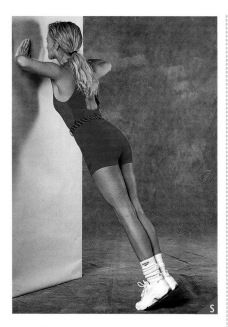 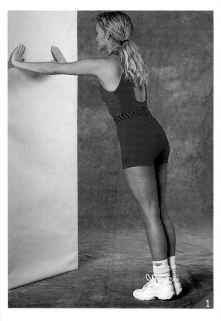

Exercise
With elbows out, shoulders pressed down, standing on the balls of her feet, Daniela extends her arms, pushing herself away from the wall. Her whole body keeps its alignment. She exhales when pushing away from the wall and inhales while returning to start.

Reps
8–16×
8–24×

Info

Keep the hands and arms wider than shoulder width, otherwise you will be training your triceps muscles more than chest.

Info

The further away you are from the wall, the more difficult the exercise will be.
Make sure you keep your ab muscles pulled together.
In this way, you won't fall into a swayback.

Tip

This exercise is ideal for pregnant women or for those who are more than 40 pounds overweight.

11. Standing Chest Stretch

Starting Position
Stand in a neutral position, legs slightly bent and upper body lifted. The head is relaxed and shoulders pressed down.

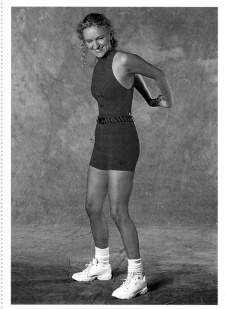

Exercise
As Daniela is demonstrating, clasping hands together behind the back, raise both arms up without leaning forward, and extend them. Inhaling, she lifts and expands her chest. As she exhales, she lifts and extend her arms just a little more. Hold 20–30 seconds.

Tip

Remember to keep your back straight during this exercise.
Also make sure that you don't extend your head forward while stretching.

12. One-Arm Chest Stretch

Starting Position
Start by standing facing a wall. Lift your right arm up and place it against the wall, then turn and place your feet *parallel* to the wall.

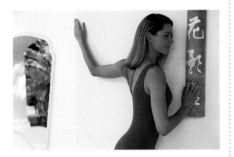

Exercise
Position the foot that is closer to the wall slightly forward, both feet point-ing forward. Adjust the arm that is on the wall so you feel a pulling in the chest muscle, *not in the front part of your shoulder!* Keeping the arm in position, now gradually turn your body away from the wall. You should feel a nice pulling sensation where your chest muscle is. Hold 20–30 seconds.

Info

The chest muscle is one of the tightest muscles in the body. Always stretch it after training.

Tip

For those with very poor posture—
stretch, stretch, stretch
your chest. And work
your upper-back muscles.
You should train in a 3-to-1 ratio:
three back exercises to
one chest exercise.

13. Seated Chest Stretch

Starting Position
Loren shows you the starting position for exercise 11 in a seated position. As you see, she is holding her back absolutely straight.

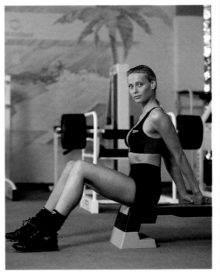

Exercise
Your arms start low, shoulders pressed down. Slowly raise your arms as far as you can without leaning forward. Hold 20–30 seconds.

Tip

Hold your arms in the starting
position and pull them downwards
and you will have a good stretch
for the front shoulder muscles.
Keep your back straight, especially
as you pull your arms upwards.
Be careful not to fall into
a swayback.

14. Chest Stretch on the Floor—Partners

Starting Position
Maria and Amanda are sitting back to back with their legs crossed. Maria leans onto Amanda's back, as Amanda leans forward.

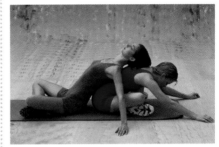

Exercise
Maria stretches her arms out, opening her chest. In this relaxed position she can achieve an optimal stretch.
After 20 to 30 seconds, Amanda will take her turn stretching her chest muscles. Hold 20–30 seconds.

Info

The pectoral muscles are normally
very tight. It is extremely important
to stretch them after exercising
this muscle group.
The partner that is leaning forward
is stretching the gluteal muscles!

Tip

To get the full benefit of this
chest stretch, inhale and exhale
deeply and try to relax into
the stretch.

Arms

Strengthen Biceps

and Triceps

We need the muscles that bend and extend our arms for everyday tasks. With goal-oriented exercise for these muscle groups, we can make many jobs a lot easier.

Exercises for the Biceps

In daily living, our biceps muscles are used far more often than our triceps muscles: to carry packages, groceries, and small children, for example. The muscle itself is easy to recognize.

Every time you pick something up or you pull something toward you, you are working your biceps muscles. The biceps brachii is that somewhat bulging fleshy muscle on the front of the upper arm that extends from the two tendons covering your shoulder blade, runs along the front of your arm, and attaches at the front of your elbow. Another muscle in this group is the brachialis, which lies under the biceps and also helps to bend the arm.

Both of these muscles help to bend your arm at the elbow. The biceps also pull your arm forward at the shoulder and turn your forearm outward. When you pull a chair across the room or pick up and carry a child, these are the muscles that are doing the major portion of the work.

Technique Tips for Biceps Exercises

❶ **Try to isolate these muscles when training. This means keeping the body very stable and just using the arms when lifting the forearm upwards.**

❷ **Be careful to keep your wrist in a neutral position, in order to avoid injury to the wrist joint or lower arm. One should not try to train upper and lower arm muscles at the same time.**

❸ **Don't overestimate your strength. It is far more effective to begin with less intensity and/or resistance and build up slowly. If you choose resistance that is too heavy, you run the danger of using your back to perform the exercise. "Falling" into a swayback position can result in injury to your spine.**

❹ **Remember to exhale when contracting the muscle and inhale during the release phase.**

❺ **Keep the elbow in its stabilized position throughout the exercises.**

❻ **Don't allow the forearm to completely close into the upper arm. When this happens the muscle is no longer contracting efficiently. On the other hand, don't allow the arm, i.e., the elbow, to hyperextend when returning to the starting position. Remember to tense the muscles when lowering the arm and to stop just before the elbow is extended.**

1. Unilateral Biceps Pull-Ups

Starting Position
Debbie is standing with bent legs, one slightly in front of the other. Her front foot is anchoring the tubing. Her arms are bent at a 90-degree angle and her forearms are held at her waist. She holds the tubing handles with her palms turned upwards and wrists in an absolutely neutral position.

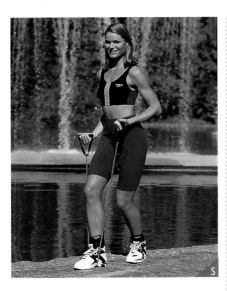 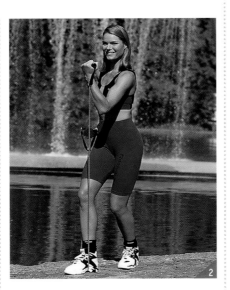

Step 1
Keeping her right arm in a 90-degree angle, Debbie lifts the tubing. The movement is slow and fluid. The elbow rises no more than shoulder height. Slowly lower arm to starting position.

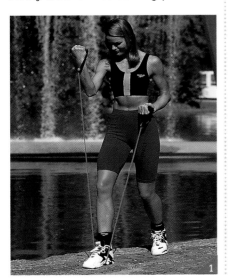

Step 2
Repeat Step 1 with the left arm.

Reps
⬤▬⬤ 4–8× per arm
⬤▬⬤ 8–16× per arm

Tip
This exercise is a challenge technically. I recommend bending the hands slightly towards you in order to protect your wrists. For advanced readers, try standing in a narrow squat position, both feet anchoring the tubing. Don't fall backwards as you pull up on the tubing. *Standing with your back to a wall would be a good reminder to stand straight.*

2. Bilateral Bicep Pull-Ups with Tubing

Starting Position
Take the same starting stance as in exercise 1. Your arms are bent at a 90-degree angle and held at waist height.

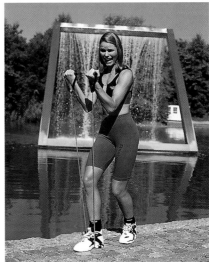

Exercise
Keeping the arms in the 90-degree angle, raise the arms together, as a unit, upwards slowly until the elbows are parallel to the shoulders. Using a lot of control, lower the arms, again as a unit, to their starting position. As you raise and lower the arms, pull your abdominal muscles together and make them very tight. In this way, you not only stabilize but train them.

Reps
⬤▬⬤ 4–8×
⬤▬⬤ 8–16×

Variation
Right arm, raise & lower 4-8
Both arms, raise & lower 4-8×
Left arm, raise & lower 4-8×
Both arms, raise & lower 4-8×

3. Biceps Curls with Bodybar

Starting Position
Stance is neutral, knees slightly bent. Fix elbows at the waist, your forearms extending in front of your thighs. Hold the bodybar with neutral wrists.

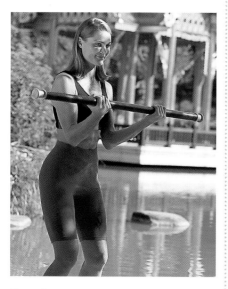

Exercise
Debbie shows effective forearm height. Do bodybar movements slowly and with control. Lower back to start position.

Reps
 Use pole 8–16× (slowly, with muscles tight)
With bodybar or dumbbell 8–20×

Variation
Use tubing, see ex. 1,2 for stance. Beginners: 4–8× light tubing; middle/advanced: 8–16× mid to heavy tubing.

Tip
Keep wrists neutral; trunk and upper body stable. *Don't* lean back. Start with resistance for good technique, and increase gradually.

4. Concentration Curls over a Chair Back

Starting Position
Sit backwards in a chair with a back that comes just under your arm. Extend your working arm over the chair back and press slightly into the inside of your thigh. In this position, we can isolate the bicep muscles better, use less assistance from the deltoid muscle. Press shoulders down during the exercise.

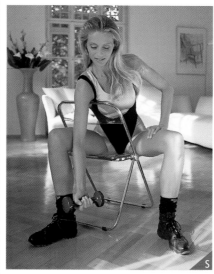
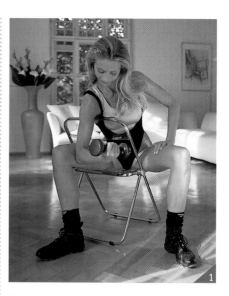

Exercise
With a slow, continuous movement raise your forearm. Tense your arm muscles through the entire exercise. With the same tempo and tension lower the arm to start position. Exhale when curling, inhale when extending.

Reps
Weights up to 4 lbs., 4–12×; repeat other arm
Weights over 5 lbs., 8–20×; repeat other arm

Info
Make sure you press your upper arm into the inside of your thigh—this helps stabilize your arm, which enables you to work your biceps more specifically.

Tip
Sit up straight and lean slightly into your working side. Bend the arm only as far as Loren shows you here, insuring effective contraction of biceps muscles. Remember to choose the right weight for yourself—if it is too heavy you'll use momentum to perform the exercise—and that isn't effective training.

5. Concentration Curls on a Step

Starting Position

Sit on the edge of a step, extend your working arm, and press the upper part of it against your inner thigh. Keeping your back straight, lean into the working side. Your other arm is bent and your hand rests on your thigh. Hold weight with neutral wrists. Keep shoulders down at all times.

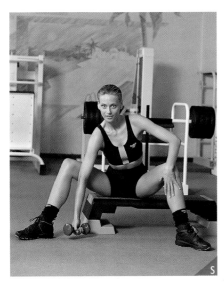 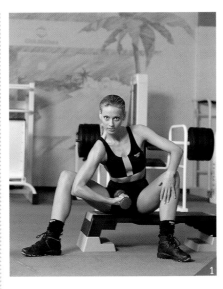

Exercise

When bending your arm, bring your forearm inward (*not* in front and upward as in exercise 4). You want to end up with your palm facing the ceiling. When bringing your arm back to the starting position, *don't over-extend* (hyperextend) the elbow and don't put the weight down on the floor during the exercise. If you can barely finish your last rep, let your other arm assist you by holding your working forearm on the outside.

Reps

Weight up to 4 lbs. 4–12×; repeat with other arm
Weight over 5 lbs. 8–20×; repeat with other arm

Tip

Always think about keeping your wrist neutral.
Although you lean into the working arm, keep your back straight throughout the exercise.
Exhale with the curl, exhale with the extension.
Your choice of weight should allow for good technique. Also, be careful: if it's too heavy, you could compromise your back.

6. Double-Duty Biceps/Triceps with Rubber Bands

Starting Position

Legs are flexed and just over shoulder-width apart. Amanda holds band with one palm up, one down. Arms are close to body, elbows at waist.

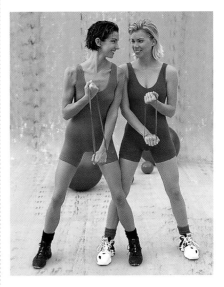

Exercise

Maria pulls rubber band in opposite directions. Arm with palm upwards pulls band upwards, working the bicep muscles; arm with palm down presses band downwards with the forearm, working the tricep. During the whole exercise, arms remain steady.

Reps

8–12× light tubing; change arms
8–20× mid to strong tubing; change arms

Tip

Keep neutral posture
In order to keep wrist stable, curl working hands toward inside of your forearm.
Press shoulders down.

Exercises for the Triceps

If you are female, beware. The state of your triceps can reveal your age. If you wave goodbye and stop, but your triceps don't, well...it's time to exercise this small but revealing body part. Even if it doesn't get close to actually "waving," a firm triceps muscle is your best bet for youthful, well-toned upper arms.

If you watch men and women exercising, you might notice the men working hard on their upper bodies with heavy free weights whereas the majority of women either choose only lower body exercises or extreme light resis-tance, if any, for upper body work. Most women fear building too much muscle and looking masculine. This, of course, is nonsense. Well formed, defined arms look athletic or just healthy and youthful, depending on the muscle make-up of your arms and how you have exercised them. My models will not go anywhere without their tubing or rubber bands. Many of them even use heavy free weights or barbells when working out. None of my models look masculine and they all have more modeling jobs than many others because they look healthy!

The muscles responsible for the outside of the upper arm are the triceps brachii with its three upper tendons, one attached to the shoulder blade, the other two on the back of your arm bone. The triceps are responsible for arm extension. When you push a cupboard door closed, push down on a bicycle pump or push yourself up from a lying position, you are using your triceps muscles.

When using your biceps, your triceps muscles are working antagonistically. They are the agonist to the biceps when they are doing the active work. Because of this, all biceps technique tips apply to the triceps exercises as well.

Important Technique Tips for Triceps Exercises

❶ If you are new to exercise, pick out triceps exercises that are easier to perform. Try to isolate the muscles. This means you are capable of performing the exercise without using momentum or moving your trunk or upper body.

❷ Remember to stabilize your elbows and just extend the lower arm. Shoulders should be pressed down, your wrist should constantly be held in a neutral position. (Think of your hand as an extension of the lower arm.)

❸ Certain positions make the exercise more difficult, so always begin with less weight or resistance and build up in each position. If you misjudge your capabilities and overload too soon, you're in for set-backs—and we don't want that!

❹ Remember to exhale when contracting your muscles. This means upon extension of the arm. Inhale when returning your arm to its start position.

❺ Be very careful *not* to swing your arms back and forth. Think of your starting and ending position as the letter "L" tipped over on its side.

1. Triceps Dip
(a classic exercise)

Starting Position
Slide off bench, back parallel to support. Press shoulders down. Place feet beyond knees (knees over/ behind heels). Bend elbows to lower body.

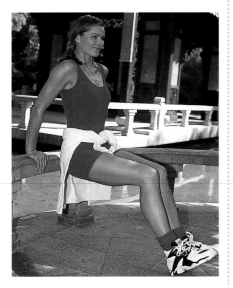

Exercise
Without raising shoulders, push up by extending arms. Keep body absolutely stable. Return to start position slowly.

Reps
⊂━⊃ 4–8×
⊟⊟ 8–16×

Variation
For very advanced, place bodybar or dumbbell in hip/thigh crease.

Tip

Keep back straight; don't move hips forward at push-up. If wrists are weak, make fists and use padding. For more resistance, use bodybar or dumbbells (variation above) or extend legs, but keep back straight and parallel for support.

2. Unilateral Triceps Kickbacks—Kneeling

Starting Position
Kneel with one leg on a bench or step, the other leg should be in a 90-degree angle, your knee over or behind your heel. Stabilize your position with your supporting arm. Your working arm is bent in an L position and is placed close to your body. Your back is long and straight.

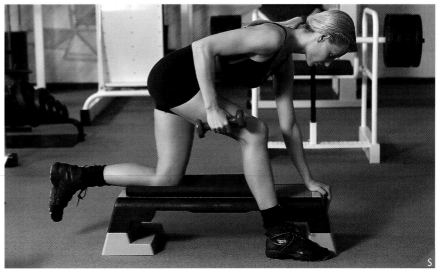

Exercise
Holding your elbow absolutely still, slowly extend your lower arm backwards. Keep your arm close to your body, your back very straight, hips parallel to floor, and abs pulled inwards. Your neck and head are building a flat line with your back. Your back should be so flat that you could use it as a tray! Return your arm to its starting position with lots of control and remember to keep the arm in an L shape!

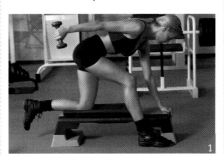

Reps
⊂━⊃ 8–12×, freeweight up to 3 lbs., change arms
⊟⊟ 8–12×, freeweight up to 8 lbs., change arms (up to 3 sets)

Tip
Make sure the knee on the step is directly under your hip; like the front leg, it too should be in a 90-degree angle.
Isolate the movement by working only from the elbow joint.
Don't swing your body.
Keep your wrist in an absolutely neutral position.

3. Standing Bilateral Triceps Kickbacks with Tubing

Starting Position

Amanda is in a starting, neutral stance. Tubing winds around her waist from back to front, crosses, then to back again. Arms form an upside-down L.

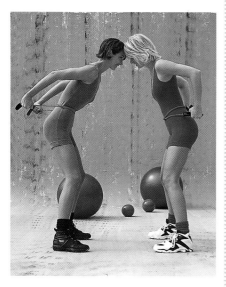

Exercise

Maria holds the tubing, not the handles, to keep tension in the tubing throughout the exercise. She extends her forearms straight back behind her, keeping elbows fixed in place. Slowly, she returns to the starting position; the tension remains in the tubing.

Reps

4–8×; without tubing 16–32×
8–12×

Tip

Lean slightly forward with your upper body and hold this position throughout the exercise.
If you can't wind the tubing around your waist twice, just place it in front; hold it so it has the correct tension.

4. Seated Triceps Extension with Tubing

Starting Position

Loren has looped one end of the tubing around a chair leg, anchoring it with the weight of the stool so it won't slide up. Her working arm holds the tubing (not the handle) and is bent backward with elbow pointing forward, an upside-down L. The palm of her hand faces inward. Loren's non-working arm rests in her lap.

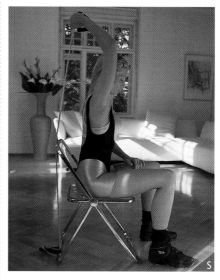 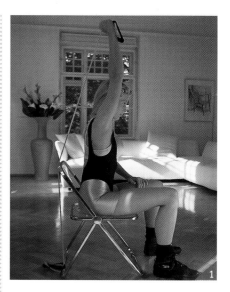

Exercise

Without moving her elbow, Loren pulls the tubing by extending her arm towards the ceiling. The arm should be almost completely extended before lowering it slowly to the starting position. Remember to exhale while the arm is on its way up and exhale on the downward movement.

Reps

4–16×, maximum of 3 sets; change arms

Info

This is a difficult exercise. If you cannot master the technique with tubing, use hand weights.
This exercise is best performed in a sitting or supine (lying on your back) position, thus keeping the back stabilized.

Tip

Be careful to slightly round the wrist by bending your hand inward and then stabilizing it. (This helps you to work against gravity.)
Keep this position throughout the exercise.
Keep your trunk absolutely stable. Remember to control the resistance; don't start off with the tubing too short.

5. Lying Triceps Extensions with Bodybar

Starting Position
Loren is in a supine position on an inclinedstep adjusted to level three at head, level one at bottom. Her legs are bent and knees placed shoulder-width apart. She holds the bodybar with a narrow grip (about a head's width apart). The backs of her hands face the step; her elbows point to the ceiling.

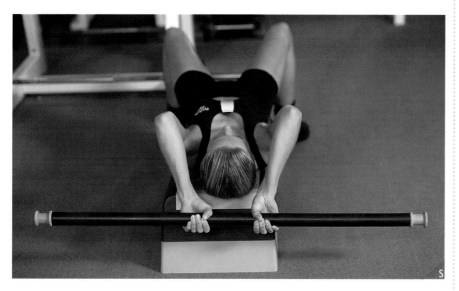

Exercise
Loren now extends her forearms to the ceiling but *without* moving her elbows forward. They remain fixed in the starting position. The forearms are returned slowly to the starting position. Remember your breathing during this exercise. Think about exhaling while extending the arms and at the same time pulling the abdominals tight, and pressing them in towards your backbone—thus stabilizing your back.

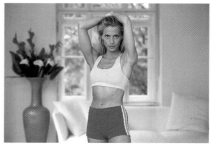

Reps
 8–12× with a pole
8–12× with a bodybar or dumbbell (maximum 3 sets)

Because this exercise is technically difficult, choose a lighter weight to insure proper technique.

Tip
Keep wrists neutral.
Be very careful to keep elbows fixed; only the forearms move.
When returning to start position, keep the L-angle of the arms. Don't open the elbows, i.e., don't let them fall sideways.

6. Triceps Stretch

Starting Position
Loren stands in a neutral position with one arm bent behind her head. The fingertips should touch the opposite shoulder blade.

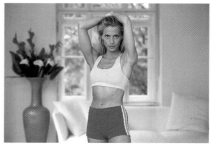

Exercise
The other hand grasps the bent arm on the back of the upper arm just above the elbow and pulls it gently toward the middle of the back.
Hold the arms close to the body.
It is important to relax the shoulder area as much as possible. Remember to breathe properly. If you push your head slightly against your bent arm, you can intensify the stretch. Hold 20–30 seconds.

Tip

If you lean slightly into the direction you are pulling, you will get a nice stretch for your latissimus as well.

Back

Good Posture—The Key

to Strength

In the beginning, man stood up and walked on two feet. The construction of the human back is a small work of mechanical genius. Unfortunately, it is also one of our number one problem areas!

Exercises for the Upper Back

Although most people believe that the stomach or the thighs are the number one problem area of the body, they are mistaken—sorely mistaken. The back is the body part that causes even so-called healthy people much distress. In our daily lives, we seldom really use our back or stomach muscles. Because of this, they are weak, and because of their weakness, many of us suffer from back problems...even very young people do!

"Sit up straight!" "Pull your shoulders back!" Do you remember your mother saying those words to you? Her advice used to get on our nerves, but she was oh so right! The construction of the human body can be compared to that of a house; each has its own statics governing equilibrium. The stability of the whole body is dependent on strong trunk muscles. If the statics in a house is not stable, with time the house will sag and eventually the walls will crack. It's the same principle with the human body. The spine and all its connecting muscles hold us up and allow us to walk. The upper back consists of many muscles; the largest is the M. latissimus, the V-shaped muscle. Someone who has what is called a "broad back," has a well-developed "lat" muscle.

Our neck is formed from the M. trapezius muscle. This muscle has three parts: the upper or ascending muscle of the trapezius, the middle section, and the lower section that runs horizontally along the upper back. Underneath the trapezius lie the rhomboid muscles, which are partially responsible for pulling the shoulder blades together. When you sit slouched, with a rounded upper back, these muscles are in a "stretched" or lengthened state. If you are constantly in this position, these muscles lose their muscle tone and become very weak, unable to pull or hold the shoulder blades together. You then have a chronically rounded back.

There are a multitude of small muscles responsible for the cervical and thoracic areas. If the main muscles are weak, then the smaller muscles are also affected. Through the stress of our daily lives, the muscles in our necks and upper backs are not only weakened, they also become stiff. This means that muscle strength training goes hand in hand with stretching to insure the optimal flexibility of these body parts. If you sit for long sessions, take a break at least every 30 minutes. Roll your shoulders backward in small circle-like movements. Pull your shoulder blades together and hold them for about a count of 8 in this position, then rub them together. I call this "self massage." Keep your shoulders pressed down during these exercises. Tip your head over to one side, hold for a count of 8, then change sides. These small "mobilization" exercises really help tone up the muscles and get the circulation functioning in those areas.

Technique Tips for Upper-Back Exercises

❶ **Perform every exercise with slow and controlled movements.**
❷ **Always keep the head in a straight line with the spine, so you don't compress the neck vertebrae.**
❸ **Keep your abdominal muscles pulled together at all times. Remember that the back and abdominals are partner-muscle groups.**
❹ **Keep your shoulders depressed while exercising. Don't let your head retract like a turtle's!**
❺ **Keep your trunk very still; if the instructions call for sitting with a straight back, keep it straight during the whole exercise.**
❻ **Don't forget your breathing technique; to exhale when you contract your muscles and inhale when you release or relax.**

1. Static and Dynamic Strengthening—Seated with a Pole

Starting Position
Sit very straight in chair, feet flat on floor or as Daniela has hers. The pole is held above the head and slightly foreward; arms are partially bent.

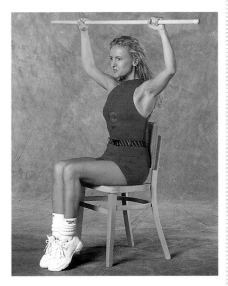

Exercise 1 (static)
Hold pole tightly. Try to pull hands away from each other, without actually moving them. Hold tension to a count of 8 or 10. Then relax; breath in, then out. Now, grasping pole tightly again, pull hands towards each other. Again, hold for an 8 or 10 count. Repeat 3×.

Exercise 2 (dynamic)
Pull pole down to sternum, do first static movement (i.e., pulling hands *away*) above. Then, slowly bring the pole upwards and repeat, for your first set. The second set is performed with hands pulling towards each other.

Reps
⊂▭ 8–12×, 2 sets
⊟ 8–16×, 3 sets

Static hold to count of 8–10 seconds.

2. Standing Lat Pull with Tubing

Starting Position
Stand in neutral position, legs apart at shoulder width. Hold tubing tautly over and slightly forward of head. From the beginning, make sure wrists are neutral.

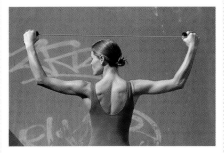

Exercise
Slowly pull elbows down and slightly towards the back, directing tubing to your sternum (like on a fitness center lat pull machine). Slowly return tubing to start position.

Reps
⊂▭ 4–12×, 2 sets
⊟ 8–24×, 3 sets

Info

Remember to stabilize upper body. Don't fall backward when pulling down tubing—a classic mistake with lat pulls on machines.

Tip

For more stability, do exercise while seated, or stand in a small lunge (see bicep ex. 1, p. 59). Toughies may double tubing and perform 8–12 reps for 3 sets. Don't forget breathing technique.

3. Standing Unilateral Lat Pulls with Tubing

Starting Position
Same as exercise 2. Hold one end of tubing over and forward of middle of your head; the other arm to side at slightly above shoulder height.

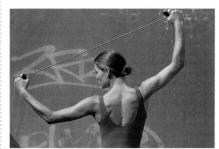

Exercise
The arm that is over the middle of your head will remain stable; the other arm directs the tubing downward by pulling the elbow down sideways and slightly to the back. Bring the tubing slowly back to start. Make sure that you control the tubing at all times. Your movements should be slow, controlled, and fluid.

Reps
⊂▭ 4–12×, 2 sets; change arms
⊟ 8–24×, 3 sets; change arms

Tip

Remember that the upper arm is responsible for creating resistance. Keep it rock steady! Because of the statically held arm, you are also working the shoulder muscles.

4. Lat Pulls with Partner

Starting Position

Amanda stands behind Maria with her legs slightly more than shoulder-width apart. She maintains a neutral posture throughout the exercise. Maria sits very straight, shoulders pressed down. Her arms are extended but slightly bent as she holds Amanda's hands.

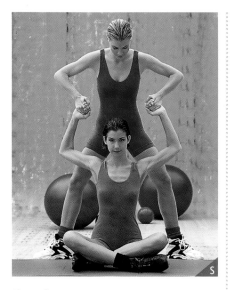 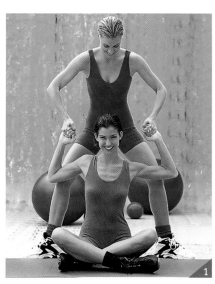

Exercise

Maria tries to pull her arms downward as Amanda offers just enough resistance to make it a little difficult. Maria should perform the movement slowly and fluidly. If Maria can't move her arms downward, then Amanda has to reduce the resistance. As Maria pulls her arms down, she exhales.

Variation

If Maria offers the resistance and Amanda must pull her arms upwards, then Amanda will be doing the active muscle work.

Reps

⊂▭⊃ 8–12×
⊂▭⊃ 8–16×

Don't forget, change partner positions!

Info

This exercise can also be performed statically. Amanda makes the resistance stronger, so Maria cannot move her arms but instead pulls for 8–10 seconds and relaxes without releasing.

Tip

Keep your knees slightly bent throughout the exercise. This way you won't stress your back.

5. Double-Duty Partner Rows

Starting Position

Amanda lies prone on 1/3-declined platform, forearms on floor, head neutral, knees at angle. Tubing wraps front, back, then front; ends are even.

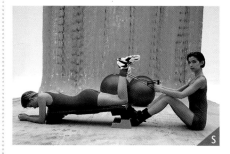

Exercise

As Amanda bends her legs towards her buttocks, Maria pulls her elbows back along sides, pinching the shoulder blades together. Slowly she returns to the start position.

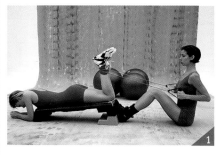

Reps

⊂▭⊃ 8–16×, change partner positions
⊂▭⊃ 8–24×, change partner positions

Tip

Prone partner can pull legs back and hold, creating more tension. Keep tubing taut throughout. Sitting partner must not bend back forward on return to start.

6. Double-Duty High-Angle Rowing with a Partner

7. Seated Low Rowing with Tubing

Starting Position

Maria's forward leg is angled, knee well behind heel. Her clasped hands hold tubing handles. Amanda stands neutrally, arm in L holds tubing taut.

Starting Position

Loren is sitting on the chair, leaning slightly forward. This lean emanates from her hips, not her back which is very straight. She's placed the tubing around one foot in a footwrap. Her arms are slightly bent, the backs of her hands are facing forward (thumbs in toward body).

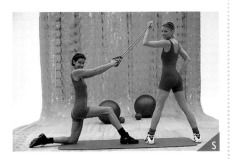

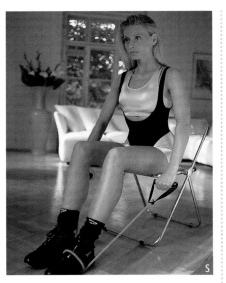

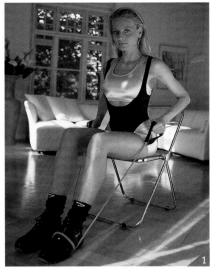

Exercise

As Amanda slowly raises her working arm upwards, Maria pulls her elbows down and backwards, close to the sides of her body. As she pulls, her body remains in the starting position.

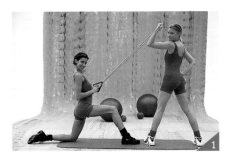

Exercise

Loren pulls the elbows back along the sides of her body, turning her hands outwards (thumbs up). When doing this exercise be careful to keep the wrists neutral, the shoulder blades pulled together and the shoulder blades depressed.

Reps

8–16×, 3 sets
8–24×, 3 sets

Reps

For advanced exercisers *only*: this exercise not for beginners. 8–24×; change positions

Info

The fixed point of resistance is coming from above.
Amanda is training her shoulder muscles and Maria her M. latissimus.

Tip

Really concentrate on pulling your shoulder blades together.

Tip

The point of resistance is coming from below.
Keep your body very straight and rock steady.
Don't lean forward when you are pulling back.
The feet must be kept flat on the floor.
If the tubing doesn't offer you enough resistance, attach the footwrap around both feet.

8. Kneeling Unilateral Row with Hand Weight

9. Prone Back Flies

Starting Position

Place a knee on a bench or platform, and the other leg so the knee is over or behind the heel. Keep back long and flat, extend arm by floor leg.

Starting Position

You may use either a flat or inclined platform (3/1) or bench. The elbows are held shoulder height, slightly bent with elbows back, palms inward. The head is held free of the platform and in line with the back. The tips of the toes are on the floor, abs and buttocks are squeezed tightly.

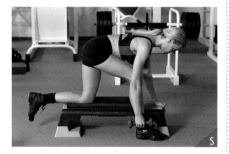

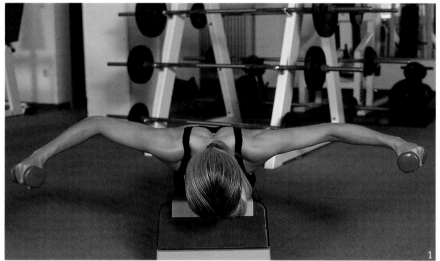

Exercise

Loren slowly raises elbow in direction of ceiling, pulling shoulder blade to the middle of her back. Slowly she lowers her arm to the start position.

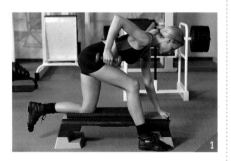

Exercise

Raise arms towards ceiling, keeping them in set position. Your palms naturally face the floor. Do not move chest or upper body as you raise your arms, but squeeze your shoulder blades together. Try to keep both arms aligned parallel to your shoulders to really work your trapezius muscles. Lower the weights but don't actually set them down on the floor. Tension should remain in your muscles even in the resting position between lifts. Perform the exercise *slowly*.

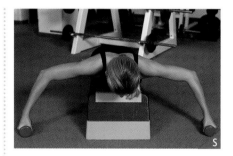

Reps

Depending on amount of weight lifted,
8–12×, 2 sets
8–24×, 3 sets

Reps

4–12×, without weights first few sessions
8–16×, 3 sets

Info

Loren lifts 6 lbs. Her supporting arm and back leg stabilize her body.

Tip

Pull abs tight and keep back straight. Head aligns with back.

Variation

You can also perform the exercise unilaterally (one arm at a time); for example, alternating right and left arms with each lift, or doing 8 reps right then 8 reps left.

Tip

Keep eyes toward floor to align neck and back.
Even if you train often, do exercise without weights to start.
Don't pull head back during shoulder blade squeeze and raising arms.

10. Seated Back Flies with Hand Weights

Starting Position
Sit in a chair with your feet flat on the floor. Holding your arms extended down along the sides of your body, lean forward. The palms of your hands are facing inwards. Although Loren, here, is working with 6-lb. weights, the exercise should be done without weights to start and until technique is perfected.

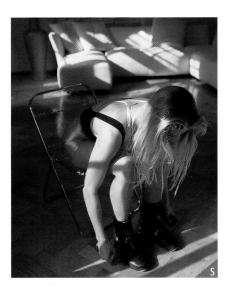

Variation
This exercise may be done unilaterally also; either the right 8× then change and do left, or alternate left and right.

Reps
8–12×
8–24×

Exercise
Raise both arms to sides, elbows leading, squeezing shoulder blades together. Exhale on up move; inhale on down. Lower slowly with control.

Tip
Do this exercise without weights, if your technique is not 100%. Also, a small pillow between chest and legs can support your trunk. Pull abs together during the entire exercise.

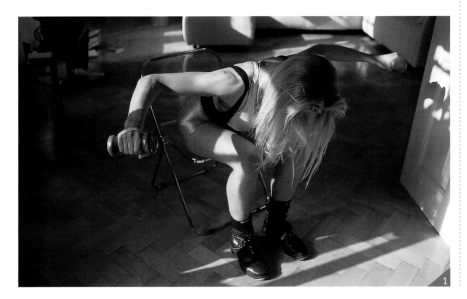

11. Bow and Arrow with Rubber Bands

Starting Position
Amanda and Maria both stand in wide lunge, toes facing front. The rubber band is held like a bow. The backs of the hands face upward (palms down).

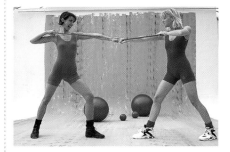

Exercise
Maria pulls the bent arm further back as if she were cocking a bow. The shoulder blade of the working arm is pulled to the middle of the body. The elbow leads the movement. The palms are down and the wrists are kept absolutely neutral. Slowly return to the start position.

Reps
8–12×; change arms
8–24×; change arms

Tip
Keep your elbow up and in line with your shoulder.
Keep your shoulders depressed throughout the exercise.
Really make sure your wrists are one line with the forearm.
Do this exercise in front of a mirror to check your technique.
Make sure the band is already taut in the starting position and keep tension in the band throughout the exercise.

12. Upright Rows with Tubing

Starting Position
Place a foot mid-tube as you stand in a narrow lunge. Lay the handles over one another and hold them both together, as Amanda is showing you.

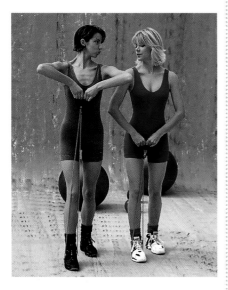

Exercise
As Maria demonstrates, keep the wrists straight and the elbows up and out. Pull upwards on the tubing so that your elbows are level with your shoulders. Pull the shoulder blades together and the exercise works the upper trapezius and shoulders as well.

Reps
⊂▭⊃ 8–12×
⊟▭⊟ 8–24×

Tip
Doing this exercise while standing against a wall, legs less than shoulder-width apart, will prevent your falling backwards as you pull the tubing upwards (a common mistake).

13. Seated Barrel Stretch

Starting Position
Grasp the back of one hand with the other. Round your arms, bringing them in front of you, as if you are holding a huge barrel!

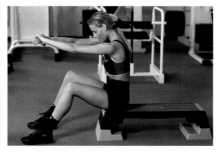

Exercise
Pull your shoulder blades away from one another and really open up your upper back. Let your head sink down slightly and pull your chest in. You should feel a pleasant stretching of the neck and upper back. Hold 20–30 seconds.

Info
Our muscles become unbalanced because of how we live, the things we do or don't do, or the sports we play. They are imbalanced when one muscle group is disproportionately stronger/tighter/shorter than its opposing muscle group. Ideally, all the muscle groups in our body should be strong and flexible. The saying "that which you wish to strengthen must also be stretched" holds very true. Training plans should include a *balance* of strength and flexibility exercises.

14. Lat and Oblique Partner Stretch

Starting Position
Amanda and Maria stand with inside legs next to each other, the outside legs out slightly wider than shoulder width. Their outside arms are joined.

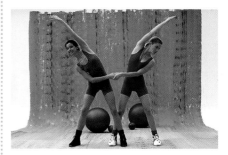

Exercise
The hands of the outside arm meet at waist height. The inside arms are extended overhead and pull the body to the side. The partners pull away from one another, creating their own point of resistance with their held hands. Hold 20–30 seconds; change sides.

Tip
Turn the palms forward and lean back just a little with the upper body; and you will feel the stretch just a bit differently. Remember to keep your knees slightly bent as you stand in the neutral position.

Info
The stretching should be felt in the upper back and waist; some will feel it right down to the top of their hips.

15. Standing Half Moon Stretch

Starting Position
Daniela stands with one leg crossed over the other, feet pressed together, knees slightly bent. Her right arm is extended above her head.

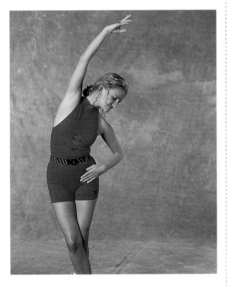

Exercise
Pull your arm farther upwards to increase the stretch. You can push your right hip slightly outwards also, to increase the stretch, but your back must remain in the neutral position. Hold 20–30 seconds; change sides.

Info

As you stretch, you may notice one side tighter or easier to stretch than the other. Stretching makes you aware of your body and its strengths and weaknesses. Learn to listen to your body. Stretch tighter sides longer and more often to achieve a balance. The same goes for muscle training.

16. Side Trunk Stretch

Starting Position
Hold onto a post or a door frame, something that is easy to grasp and won't move. Place both feet close to the object.

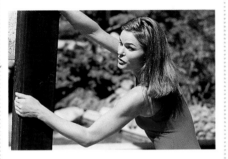

Exercise
Now, pull away from the object, leading with your hips and the side of your back. The further you pull away with your hips, the more stretch you will feel. Hold 20–30 seconds, then change sides.

Info

Flexibility is defined as the ability to perform a large range of motion over one or more joints. The goal of stretching exercises is to optimize our range of motion and at the same time strengthen joint stability.
If we apply this goal to the above exercise, then we want to stretch the right and left sections of our upper backs, but don't want to go beyond the normal range of motion in the shoulder joint.

17. Turtle Stretch for the Upper Back

Starting Position
Maria sits with her legs flexed. She bends forward, places her arms between her legs, then reaches outside each leg to grasp her ankles.

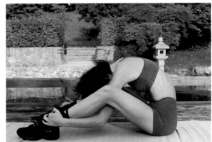

Exercise
In this position, you will pull your abs in very tightly. Now hold your ankles very tight while pulling away from them with your upper back. Open your shoulder blades by pulling them apart. Your upper back should be very rounded. Hold 20–30 seconds.

Tip

Don't forget to breathe regularly while holding your stretches (not just this one, all of them!).
Try to pull the stretch out until you have reached your limit.
It shouldn't hurt and the muscle should not start to twitch. If it does, it's time to relax and shake it out.
Be careful to come slowly out of each held stretching position.
Give your muscles a chance to return to their normal length.

Exercises for the Lower Back

The back is truly an intricate piece of engineering. Whereas the upper section of our back is responsible for and assists in the movement of our arms, shoulders and head, the entire back is like an edifice. The muscles running along the spine not only support it, thus helping us to stand erect, but also allow us to bend forward or round our entire back if we need to. These muscles are called the erector spinae and they are the principle movers of the back. They are thick, quadrilateral muscles in the lumbar region, splitting into large bundles to the ribs, upper vertebrae, neck and head in their ascent. You can usually identify these back muscles in most people.

The back is really dependent on a well-functioning muscle system. The spine with its vertebral column, vertebrae and intervertebral discs, cannot stand alone. Dozens of longer and shorter muscles, tendons and ligaments help support and stabilize this most important structure in our body. If these muscles are constantly stretched, twisted or strained due to improper movement or bad posture, while other muscles are overtrained and others not trained at all, two things could happen: At the least, you will have muscle soreness or pain, due to muscles that are too tight or tense. At the worst, you will have damage to your vertebrae or to the discs, and this could possibly lead you to the surgeon's door!

When two vertebrae are not lined up with one another, for example when you are slouching over your desk and supporting yourself with your elbows, the pressure in the spine isn't distributed evenly onto the discs, it is being absorbed by just a smaller segment of the discs. If you sit this way on a regular basis, you could damage your spine with time. The lumbar area of the spine is especially susceptible to these problems and must withstand a lot of pressure due to improper movement. Most people don't sit properly or have the correct

posture when carrying or picking up objects. Through awareness and learning to control your body and its movements through proper and goal-oriented back exercises, you can really get a "load off your back"!

Information and Technique Tips for Lower-Back Exercises

❶ **The exercises in this section are specific to the erector spinae and lumbar section of your back. It is very difficult to isolate these muscles during exercise; therefore I have offered you a series of variations that work the muscles in slightly different ways.**

❷ **Because most of these exercises are static or very slow, you might think, "Ho hum...where's the action?" Well, the action is the strength and health you will be creating in your torso! This, in turn, enables you to accomplish a lot more training for other body parts! So be consistent and include these exercises in your program.**

❸ **Remember to always pull your abs together very tight, when training your back. They are partner muscles.**

❹ **In contrast to the other exercises, you can just breathe evenly and regularly. Sometimes it is even better to inhale first when raising your upper body, exhale and then breathe evenly during the hold section of the exercise.**

❺ **Really take time when doing the stretch and relaxation exercises.**

1. Pelvic Tilt

Starting Position
Daniela is lying in a relaxed supine position with her knees bent and her legs positioned shoulder-width apart.

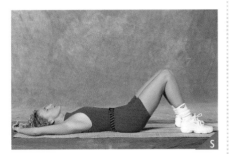

Exercise
The lower back is raised off the floor, for a "swayback," then pressed back into the floor, and the lower abdominals are contracted to bring the pelvis into a tilt. It repeats—swayback, to tilt, and back—for a rocking pattern.

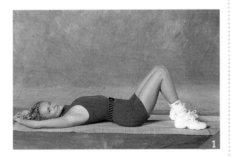

Reps
8–16×
12–32×

Tip
Keep the rocking pattern slow and fluid. Really concentrate as you do the exercise.
Practice with conscious breathing techniques: exhale on the tilt.

2. Trunk Extension (a classic exercise)

Starting Position
For this simple and classic exercise, Daniela lies face down, prone on the floor. Her hands are opened on top of each other, palms up, resting on her buttocks. Her head and neck are in line with her back. Her legs are straight, her toes touching the floor.

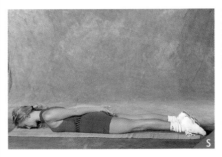

Exercise
Slowly lift head and shoulders simultaneously to the top of your chest, then lower slowly. Control your movement.

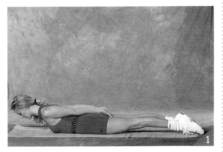

Variations
V1: Raise up a little higher, but keeping your head still in line with your back. Make sure your feet remain on the floor. Really pull your buttock muscles together.

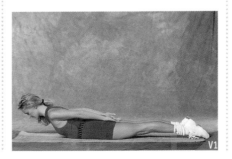

V2: For this more difficult exercise, place your hands on your forehead, elbows out. Now raise up again and slowly lower.

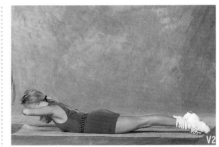

V3: For this have-a-ball variation, hold a grapefruit-sized ball (or the fruit itself!) with both hands, arms slightly rounded. Feet remain on the floor, this time in a flexed position. Pull your buttock muscles together. Raise up only slightly, bringing the arms up as well. As you raise your arms, squeeze the ball (or fruit).

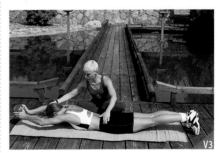

Reps
4–8×
8–12×, or lift and hold 10–20 seconds

3. Prone Leg Raise (another classic exercise)

Starting Position
Lie prone with your head relaxed and turned to the side. If you have a sway back, or you need more support, place a towel or small pad under your hips.

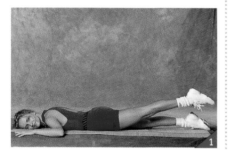

Exercise
Raise leg to feel tension in buttock and lower back. Keep leg straight and pelvis firmly on the floor (don't roll away from lifted leg). Lower slowly.

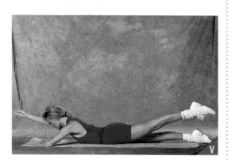

Variation
Keep head and upper back aligned; slowly raise an arm and opposite leg. Feel a "pulling" diagonally, not simply a raising movement. Tighten buttocks to stabilize. Other forearm can be used as support, but shoulders must be depressed.

Reps
- 8–12×
- 12–24×, or lift and hold 10–20 seconds; change legs and/or arms

4. Three-Point Lift (trunk stabilization)

Starting Position
Daniela is in a prone position with her arms crossed loosely on her chest. Her legs are extended and about shoulder-width apart.

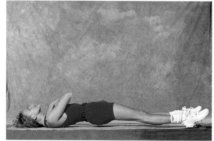

Exercise
Tighten the muscles in the trunk and buttocks. Now, raise your whole body up off the floor, leaving only the heels, shoulder blades and back of head on the floor, supporting you. Make sure you continue to breathe consistently during the holding phase of this exercise.

Reps
- Hold 10–20 seconds
- Hold 15–60 seconds

Tip

This exercise calls for a lot of concentration in order to hold your body correctly. The longer you can hold it, the stronger and more advanced you have become!

5. Opposing Arm/Leg Raise —Kneeling (balance and stabilization)

Starting Position
Your beginning stance is on all fours with your weight distributed equally over all four points. Your back is long and straight.

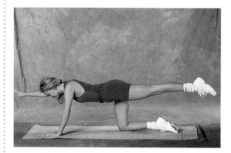

Exercise
Lift opposite arm and leg. Keep your head in line with your back and your back absolutely straight. You want to build one continuous line from front fingertip to toe. Your supporting leg forms a 90-degree angle.

Reps
- Hold 10–20 seconds
- Hold 15–60 seconds
  Change legs and arms.

Info

You should have the feeling that two people are pulling you in opposite directions—one pulling your arm, the other, your leg. Imagine your back growing longer.

Tip

Be careful not to let your upper back sink down or your midsection fall into a swayback.

6. Cat Stretch

Starting Position
Start out by getting down on all fours with your back straight.

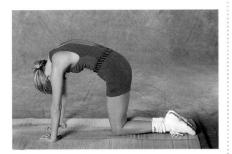

Exercise
Slowly curve your back by pulling your navel into your lower back. Really press your stomach into your lower back. It helps here to exhale when rounding the back. Slowly curve your back inwards, now inhale. Move gently up and down. If you have had back problems keep your back relatively straight when curving down.

Reps
⟨⟩ Hold 10–20 seconds
⟨⟩ Hold 15–60 seconds

Or, in motion (dynamic variation):
8–24×, moving up and down

Tip
Give yourself enough time when stretching.
This is a great exercise to do first thing in the morning.

7. Back Circles (spinal stretch and self massage)

Starting Position
Lie on your back and bring your knees to your chest. Hold lower legs just below the knees. Your entire back and head are relaxed on the floor.

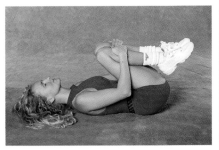

Exercise
Slowly roll your lower back in a small circle. You should feel it "massaging" the lumbar area. Roll 30 seconds to the right, then 30 seconds to the left.

Reps
As long and as often as you like!

Info
The flexibility and mobility of our back muscles is the absolute key to body balance and freedom of movement.
The spine is truly nature's work of genius as it gives us signals when we are not in balance with ourselves. These exercises have been chosen for you to improve mobility of the spine and muscular flexibility.

8. Turtle Stretch for the Lower Back

Starting Position
Maria sits with legs bent. She bends over, placing her arms between her legs then bringing them to the outside of each leg and grasping her ankles.

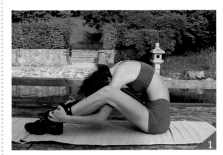

Exercise
Now, holding tightly to your ankles, pull away from them with your lower back. Slowly straighten your knees—try to press them to the floor. Push your navel into your lower back at the same time. Feel for the pull in your lower back.

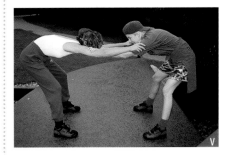

Variation
Maria and Amanda use each other to create resistance. Standing with knees bent, they grasp each other's arms. With heads down, they pull away from one another until they feel a nice stretching sensation in the lower back. Make sure that one partner doesn't pull too hard, so that you do not lose your balance. Hold the tension 20–30 seconds.

Stomach

The Center of

Our Being

Good posture is your insurance policy for a healthy back. Training the abdominals correctly and regularly is the secret to success.

Exercises for the Abdominals

The abdominal muscles are critical to good posture. Learning to train them well is a matter of communication between mind and stomach muscles.

One thing to be stressed here is that flat and well-defined stomach muscles aren't created by exercise alone. The extra fat covering them can only be successfully reduced by a combination of correct nutrition, cardiovascular exercise and, of course, efficient and effective abdominal exercises.

Here, I've brought together abdominal exercises ideal for defining and strengthening this most important part of your body. All these exercises are back and joint "friendly." You will be truly working your abdominals, not your hip flexors. If you really follow my advice and exercise your abs daily, you will be able to measure your success in just a few short weeks. The abdominal muscles tend to change structurally rather quickly. Even if you can't actually see your progress, by holding your hand against your stomach as you exercise you'll notice how hard they have become!

Over your stomach front you have four large muscles. They link the front and sides of your pelvis to the lower parts of your ribs. Arranged at different angles, they form protective sheeting over your abdominal cavity. Your abdominal muscles are arranged symmetrically on each side of the mid-line or linae alba.

Rectus abdominis forms two wide bands joining the front of your ribs to your pelvis in a vertical line. Under rectus abdominus you have two diagonally arranged muscles. The obliquus externus (external oblique) extends from your ribs to the hipbone. This muscle curves downwards and inwards. The obliquus internus (internal oblique) lies underneath the externus and runs in the opposite direction. The fourth muscle is the transversus, which lies under the other three muscles on either side of your abdomen. These muscle fibers run horizontally.

Tips for Successful Abdominal Training

❶ **Pay attention to the movement of your abs. It's those muscles that initiate each movement, and not the head, the back, or the shoulders, which simply add more resistance.**

❷ **In doing abdominal exercises, think of your stomach muscles as if they were an accordion: the last rib and your hipbone should squeeze together. If you place a thumb on your rib and middle finger on your hipbone you can feel this happen. If you have a problem coordinating this movement, here's a tip: inhale and then cough very deeply. Or, just laugh! Exhale sharply—"ha" "ha" "ha"—with no breath in-between. If you do it right, you will feel and see the thumb and middle finger move together. It takes concentration and practice, but once you master the technique you won't have to do as many reps, as you'll be training more effectively. You'll even be able to do it standing or sitting.**

❸ **Be careful, when you pull your stomach muscles together, that they are tight and don't bulge out.**

❹ **The same applies to oblique exercises: the opposite rib to hip bone, or reverse crunches, hip to rib.**

❺ **Always breathe correctly. Exhale on the contraction, inhale on the release.**

❻ **Watch out for your head. Keep it stable and about a fist-length from your collarbone (sternum). Don't pull on it when you have your hands positioned behind your head.**

1. The Crunch

Starting Position

I've asked Loren to lie in a supine position with her legs and feet flexed and aligned with her hips. Her hands are behind her head, her elbows are open. Her head is in a neutral position with her chin fist-length from her sternum, or collarbone. In this position, she lifts head and arms from the floor. The tops of her shoulder blades remain on the floor, however. Throughout the exercise, the head and arms are held in position; they are not pulled or moved.

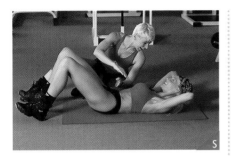

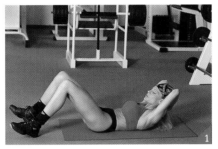

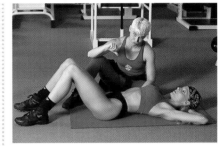

Exercise

Loren exhales, pulling lower rib into hip, contracting stomach muscles accordionlike. With upper body pulled forward, bottoms of shoulder blades and ¾s of back are on the floor. She returns slowly to starting position.

Variation

It's easier...and harder! The hands on chest, shown below, reduce resistance, so movement is easier; but the head being non-supported is hard on the neck muscles. Keep the head still and neutral throughout the exercise.

Here, Loren demonstrates a classic mistake. From this swayback position, most people will pull their heads up, closing their elbows and rounding their backs. They come up far too high, working their hip flexors instead of their abdominals. This way of working is not only inefficient, but it can cause discomfort to the back.

Tip

To relieve neck tension, place a ball the size of your fist under your chin and lightly press into it. Hold position and perform your exercise this way. It helps! Placing your feet flat on the floor also helps relax your buttocks. Don't forget to inhale before contracting, and really exhale when pulling the abs together. If your stomach tends to come up when contracting, practice pulling it *in* first, and then pulling *together* second. Be nice to your back, use a soft mat when doing crunches.

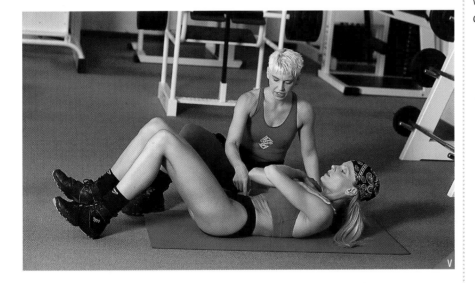

I check to see that Loren's buttock muscles are properly relaxed. It's important that the contraction come only from the abdominal muscles, not the buttocks.

Reps

8×, 2 sets
12–24×, 3 sets

2. Crunches on an Inclined Platform

Starting Position
Take the same starting position as in exercise 1, except your arms will be extended in front of you and your feet flat on the floor.

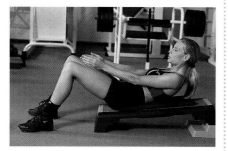

Exercise
Exhale and pull the stomach muscles together and push the arms through the legs. Keep your arms very low, the palms facing each other.

Reps
8–16×, 3 sets
16–24×, 3 sets

Variation
For advanced exercisers only, do exactly the same exercise in the decline position. Just turn around on the platform; now you will be working against gravity!

Tip
When doing crunches on the incline, make sure to keep ¾s of your back on the platform. Adjust the platform to a 3 to 1 height.

3. Ab Prayers!

Starting Position
Maria lies in a supine position, legs flexed and positioned shoulder-width apart, feet flat on the floor, and hands pressed together in front of her stomach. Her neck is long and relaxed. Maria inhales.

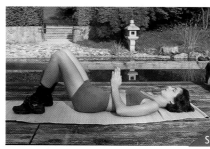

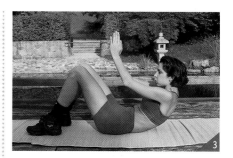

Step 1
As Maria exhales, she pulls the abdominal muscles together and rolls up. Pressing her hands together, she brings them toward the ceiling, stays in position for 2 counts, then inhales.

Step 3
Again, Maria exhales, pushing her hands together and upwards. She again holds position for a count of 2, then slowly rolls back to the starting position.

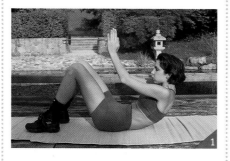

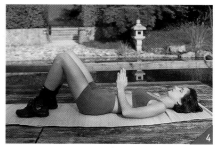

Step 2
She exhales, contracts abs more, presses hands through legs, holds to 2, inhales.

Reps
Whole sequence 4×
Whole sequence 8×; if time allows, 2 sets

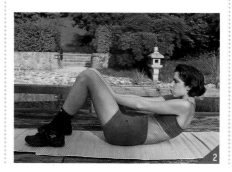

Tip
Do this exercise *slowly;* contraction should strengthen in each position. Stop and concentrate on pulling abs together. Rest between reps to reenergize before starting again.

4. Double-Duty Abs/Chest Crunch with Tubing

5. Double-Duty Abs/Chest Crunch with Hand Weights on an Inclined Platform

Starting Position
Tubing is behind our models' backs and they are holding ends. Amanda is in starting position, arms forming an L, palms facing, holding tubing taut.

Starting Position
Lie in a supine position with head on the platform, legs flexed, feet on the floor shoulder-width apart. Your arms are in an L position, upper arms are in line with your shoulders. Hold the hand weights so that your palms are facing the direction of your legs (your thumbs are inwards, pointing to each other).

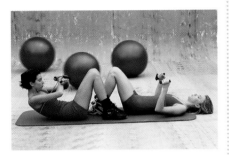

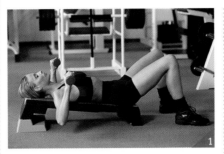

Exercise
Maria exhales, pulling her abs together, and at the same time lifts her elbows and crosses her hands in front of her chest, pulling the tubing tight. She rolls up to just below her shoulder blades, raising head and shoulders simultaneously. Then she rolls down to *almost* her starting position, but leaves head and shoulders elevated. This is her new starting position.

Step 1
Exhale, pulling abs and pressing arms together (palms facing) at the same time. Roll up, as in exercise 4. Remember to keep head and shoulders as one unit. Try not to come off platform any higher than just below shoulder blades.

Step 2
In position, inhale; now exhale and squeeze elbows and abs together. Inhale and slowly roll back to start.

If you have mastered the accordionlike technique with your abs and don't need rest in between sequences, don't roll down to starting position. As in exercise 4, roll back to just above shoulder blades and do exercise from there.

Reps
For advanced exercisers only: 8–12×, 3 sets

Reps
For advanced exercisers only: 8–12×, 3 sets

Tip
Remember to keep chin fist-length from your collarbone (sternum). Modify the exercise by not using hand weights. Or, exercise on the floor instead. Make sure that at least ¾s of your back remains flat. If strong, try using a decline bench.

Info
The tubing intensifies this exercise. You decide how much resistance to use. Don't use too much at the start or your arms will tire before your abs do.
Really curl into the movement and feel your abs pull together. Roll no higher than just below your shoulder blades.
Keep your head in neutral position.

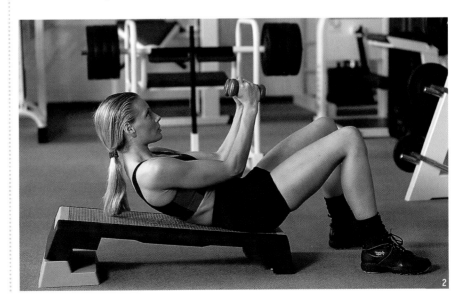

85

6. Pullover Crunch with Hand Weight on an Inclined Platform

Starting Position

Loren is in a supine position, back pressed into the platform, arms bent behind her head, both hands holding a dumbbell (or hand weight). Her legs, hips and feet are positioned as in exercise 5.

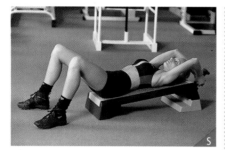 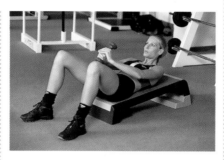

Exercise

Loren pulls her ribs towards her hips and chin slightly downward. Slowly she brings the weight over her head and down to the top of her legs. Her arms maintain the bent angle during the pullover. The movement should be controlled and fluid. Loren exhales throughout the pullover. When she rolls back, she does *not* return to start, but keeps head and shoulders slightly off platform, above shoulder blades as in exercises 4 and 5.

Reps

For advanced exercisers only: 8–16×, 3 sets

Tip

Be extremely careful *not* to fall into a swayback when you bring your arms back behind your head. If you have shoulder problems, start with weight above your head. *Don't* bring it behind your head.

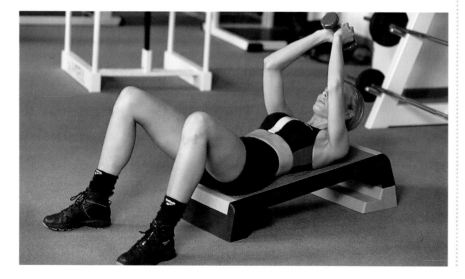

7. Reverse Crunch

Starting Position

Debbie lies with her lower legs in a 90-degree angle. She has her legs crossed (I prefer my feet side by side). Her upper body is completely relaxed.

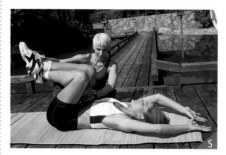

Exercise

Debbie exhales, pulling abs inward and hipbones toward ribs; this brings legs closer to the body. Her lower back, on the floor, rounds as the legs pull in.

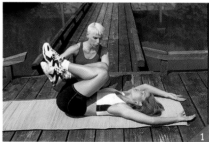

Reps

4– 8×, 2 sets
8–24×, 3 sets

Tip

Don't lift the hips—a common mistake. As you pull your legs to you, really round your back. The lower back benefits by being stretched as the abs contract. Relax your lower legs, let them rest on the back of your thighs.

8. Hip Lift on a Declined Platform

Starting Position
Extend legs straight up, knees slightly bent, feet relaxed. Grasp the sides of the step, by your head, to help you do the exercise better.

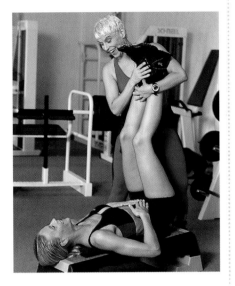

Exercise
Contract the abs and lift hips to the ceiling at the same time. Exhale as you raise yourself up. The legs stay in exactly the same starting position.

Reps
4–8×, 2 sets
8–24×, 3 sets

Tip
Don't "hop" your hips up.
Don't roll backwards, or stretch your legs up when you raise your hips.
At the start, work with a partner as I am working with Loren.
The idea isn't to come up really high, but to raise your hips properly, using the ab and back muscles.

9. Oblique Crunch

Starting Position
Lie in a supine position with legs flexed. Cross your right leg over the left one and extend your right arm. Place your left hand behind your head, open your left elbow outwards and slightly raise your left shoulder blade off of the floor.

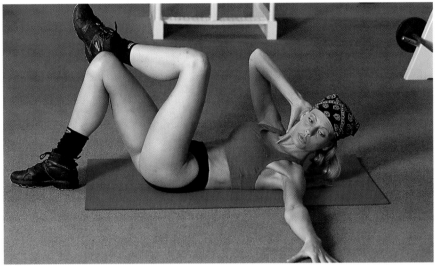

Exercise
Pull your left lower rib to your right hipbone. The "accordion" will now be working on a diagonal. As you raise up, push your left shoulder toward your right knee—your elbow stays open and out. Keep the rest of the back on the floor and your head in line with your spine, although it will naturally turn slightly into the movement. Slowly roll back to your starting position.

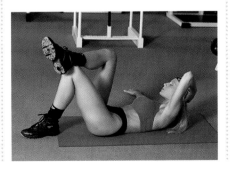

Reps
4–8×, 3 sets; change sides
8–24×, 3 sets; change sides

For beginners, it's a good idea to change sides in-between sets.

If you are advanced and want to overload, do all three sets on one side, then change.

Tip
If you can, hold your head in the neutral position without using your arm, then extend the right arm so it is on the side of the flexed thigh.
As you roll up, press it along the thigh for added resistance.
Don't forget to exhale on the contraction.

10. Partner Obliques

Starting Position
Amanda and Maria lie like bookends, buttocks to buttocks. Their legs extend upward, feet pressed against each other's for support.

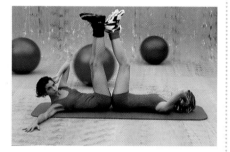

Exercise
They both do exactly the same thing as Loren did in exercise 9, except that their legs are extended and not crossed over. They initiate the movement from the rib and press it down to the hip bone, the shoulder pushing in the direction of the opposite leg and the elbow staying open and out.

Reps
⊑▭⊐ 4–8×, 2 sets; change sides
⊑▭⊐ 8–24×, 3 sets; change sides

Tip
If your hamstring muscles are very tight, save this exercise for when you have achieved the needed flexibility. Remember your breathing technique!

11. Ball Combo for Rectus and Obliques

Starting Position
Debbie has taken the supine position. Her arms are stretched out in front, down the length of her body. Her hands hold a ball the size of a grapefruit. Her head and chin are in the neutral position and they will be kept that way throughout the exercise.

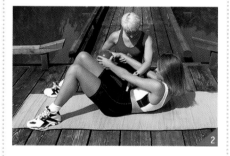

Step 1
Debbie exhales, contracting her abs like an accordion, and then pushes the ball she is holding down through her legs. She then leans back, while continuing to contract her abs, and inhales.

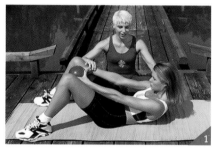

Step 2
Exhaling, she pushes ball to right, pulls rib to hipbone, and rolls back; inhales.

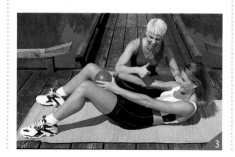

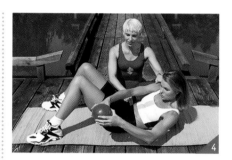

Step 3
Exhaling again, she pushes the ball through her legs, then leans back again and inhales.

Step 4
This time, she exhales and pushes the ball to the left side.

Variation
Advanced exercisers only, you can alternate pushing the ball right and left. This way you are working primarily the obliques.

Reps
⊑▭⊐ 2–4×
⊑▭⊐ 4–8×

Tip
This exercise demands real control; make each movement count. Keep the leaning back a small movement.

12. Double-Duty Oblique Lifts

Starting Position
Lie on your side with one leg on top of the other. Rest your weight on your lower arm; the other arm is in front of you to help you push up. Keep shoulders depressed. Distribute your weight so that you can stay in this side-lying position throughout the exercise.

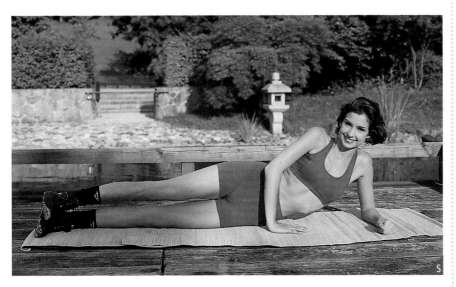

Exercise
Tense your body, exhale, and push up sideways away from the floor. Rise all the way up to the side of your shoe, keeping your legs very straight. Hold this position for about a count of 2. Inhale as you lower, but don't lower all the way down.

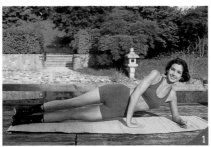

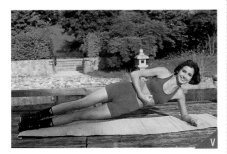

Variation
Advanced exercisers only: Place the "helping hand" on your stomach and raise up using supporting arm only.

Reps
 4–8×, 1 set
8–16×, 2 sets

Tip
This "double duty" exercise works the abductor muscles *and* on stabilizing the lower back. Make sure the legs stay extended. Really keep yourself balanced. Don't let yourself fall backwards.

13. Seated Pullbacks with Tubing

Starting Position
Sit tall; one or both feet wrapped, as desired. Hold tubing with the arms extended at your sides (absolutely straight), knuckles down.

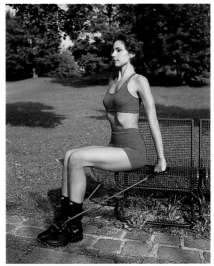

Exercise
Sit up very straight, with shoulders depressed. Exhale and pull your arms backwards along your sides. Hold for 2 count, then slowly bring arms back to your sides. You will not pull very far back; the strong tension should make that difficult. If it is done correctly, you'll feel your abs getting rock hard!

Reps
 4–8×, 2 sets
8–16×, 3 sets

Tip
To be at all effective, wrists *must* be in line with forearm. Keep shoulders depressed, and back and arms straight throughout. Really exhale when you pull arms back.

Buttocks

Firming up

....

those Buns!

....

Who wouldn't love to have nicely rounded, tight buttocks! Men and women alike find this body part very attractive in the opposite sex. But most people don't know that strong buttock muscles play an important role in good posture.

Exercises for the Buttocks

Strong, firm, well-rounded buttock muscles don't only have an esthetic value. They actually play an all-important role in our ability to move.

The buttocks are formed primarily from the large gluteus maximus. It is not only a lovely cushion when we sit, but a strong hip extensor. For example, if you climb stairs or stand up from a chair, this muscle does the majority of the work. The gluteus maximus is also responsible for helping with the adduction and abduction of our legs. It also plays a big role in rotating the leg outwards in the hip joint.

Most people don't realize that the buttocks together with the abdominals have a profound effect on the way we hold our hips; for example, if we have a swayback. The gluteals and the abdominals need to be primarily strengthened, whereas the antagonists and synergists, erector spinae and hamstrings, need to be primarily stretched, as they tend to be tight. Stretching and strengthening these partner muscle groups help correct our posture and make our backs strong. Two smaller helper muscles, the gluteus medius, located above and to the side of the gluteus maximus, and the gluteus minimus, located on the iliac crest of the hip bone, assist the gluteus maximus with rotation and abduction. For example, if you lift your leg to the side, or transfer your weight from one leg to the other, these muscles help perform these functions.

An especially effective exercise for the buttocks is the squat. This multi-functional exercise is extremely efficient because it works the hip extensors, the knee extensors, and the trunk muscles.

Technique Tips for Buttocks Exercises

❶ When lying in a supine or prone position, be careful not to lift the working leg too high. Lifting the leg higher than the buttocks puts a strain on your back and spine. Readers who have had slipped discs or other spinal problems should be most careful about following my technique guidelines. Always work in a slow and controlled manner. Lift legs; do not kick them or use momentum to raise them.

❷ Don't twist your back or lean into the supporting leg. Keep your weight in the middle and your hips parallel to the floor.

❸ Inhale on the contraction and exhale when you release.

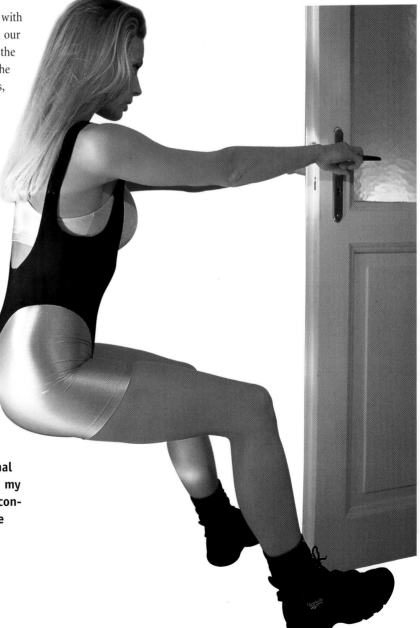

1. Prone Hip Extension

Starting Position
Lie flat on the floor—in prone position. If you have a swayback, place a small rolled-up towel under your hips for comfort. Extend the legs, but relax your foot (keep it in neutral position). Either turn your head to the side, like Daniela, or position your forehead on a pillow so that your neck and head stay in line with your back.

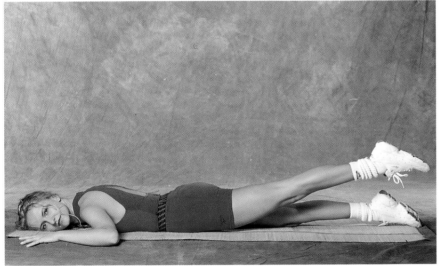

Exercise
Slowly raise extended leg until you feel your buttock tightening. Slowly lower, but don't set it back down on floor. This way, you maintain tension in the leg throughout the exercise.

Variation
Do this exercise with a bent leg as well (see ex. 2). You won't have as large a range of motion as in exercise 2, but it is easier on the knees and you can't cheat—your hips must stay on the floor!

Reps
8–24×; change legs
8–32×, or 8–12× with weights or rubber bands, 3 sets; change legs

Tip
Advanced exercisers can place a weight (1–4 lbs) behind the knee, as in exercise 2. Or, done with an extended leg, use a rubber band.

Tip
Remember to keep your foot in a neutral position. Try to consciously relax the non-working leg. To work your adductors a little more, turn your foot inward. If you want to work your buttocks a little differently, turn your foot outward.

2. Kickbacks

Starting Position
On all fours (forearms/knees), head in line with back. Place a weight (1–4 lbs.) behind a bent knee. Pull abs tight. Keep back straight, don't let yourself *sag* in the middle.

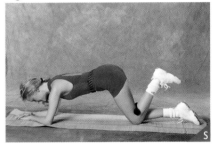

Exercise
Slowly raise the bent leg to hip height or just below; now lower it slowly but don't put it on the floor. Exhale while raising, inhale while lowering.

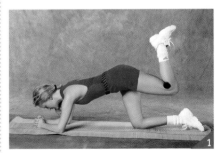

Reps
4–12×
8–12×, 3 sets
Rep number depends on weight used

Tip
Don't raise leg over hip height; if you're "tipping," it's *too high*! Keep leg lower, hips parallel to floor. Divide your weight evenly. Don't lean into the supporting leg. Test your weight distribution by raising the arm of supporting leg.

3. Supine Hip Raises with Pole

Starting Position

Lie with legs flexed a hip-width apart, heels on floor, toes raised. Pull your legs in and raise buttocks slightly off the floor. Press the pole to your hips.

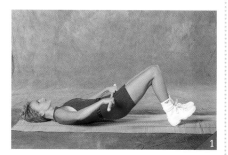

Exercise

Press hips against the stick, raising up slightly higher, and squeeze your buttocks together. Slowly lower to start position. Keep back ¾s on floor.

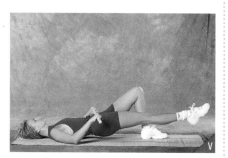

Variation

Advanced only, place foot of flexed leg flat on the floor and extend other leg, keeping a neutral foot. Now, *without* lifting extended leg, raise hip of bent leg until buttocks come slightly off the floor. Your extended leg acts like a weight during hip lifts, but only if it is kept level. Slowly lower to start, keeping leg extended. Change legs.

Reps

▱ 4–12×
▰ 8–12×

4. Prone Hip Extension on an Inclined Platform

Starting Position

Lie prone on (3/1) inclined platform, knees just off platform, toe tips on floor, head free of platform, forearms on floor. Loren uses 2-lb. ankle weights.

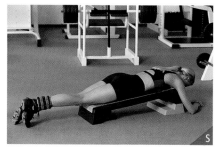

Exercise

Slowly raise extended leg until your buttock muscles contract. For more efficiency, tense buttocks before the leg raise. Lower leg, but not to floor.

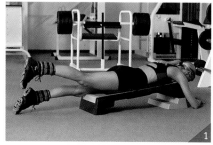

Reps

▱ With ankle weights, 4–8×; without, 8–16×; change legs
▰ With ankle weights, 8–12×, 3 sets; without weights, 12–32×; change legs

Info

The platform position gives you more range of motion in the leg. At the same time, it's easy on the knees, head and arms.

5. Door Squats

Starting Position

Holding both door handles, place feet, shoulder-width apart, on either side of door. Lean back. With weight on heels, extend arms a bit and relax knees.

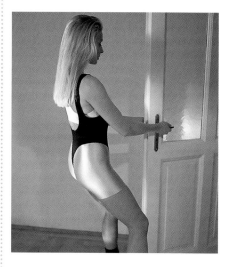

Exercise

Very slowly, sink down until buttocks are level with the knees (see Loren on page 92, large photo). Squeeze buttock muscles tightly together as you move downward. The feeling should be of going to sit in a chair a little farther back. The buttocks should remain squeezed together at all times. As the buttocks are raised upward, they should be squeezed extra hard. The upper body remains absolutely straight during the entire exercise.

Reps

Advanced or beginner:
Static: Hold in squat position 30–60 seconds, 3×
Dynamic: 8–16×, 3 sets

6. Gluteal Stretch in Supine Position

Starting Position
Lie in a prone position and bring your knees up to your chest. Rest your hands on your lower legs. Your feet are relaxed.

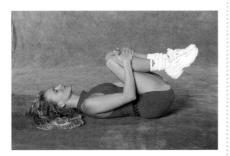

Exercise
Pull your legs in towards your chest until you feel a pleasant stretching in your buttocks. You can also place your arms in-between your lower and upper legs and pull your legs inward in that way. Hold 20–30 seconds.

Tip

For a stronger stretch, *so long as you don't have knee problems*, cross one leg over the other and pull the legs into your chest (the same as in exercise 7, but in supine position). Important: Keep your head, shoulders, and ¾s of your back on the floor.

7. Seated Gluteal Stretch

Starting Position
Do this stretch anywhere; no one will know! Cross a leg over the other *above* (not on) knee. Place hand on the foot inside of thigh. Arms are bent.

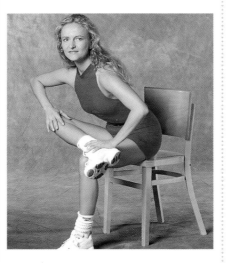

Exercise
Keeping an absolutely straight back, slowly bring your chest towards your crossed leg. The farther down you go, the greater the stretch will be; but lower yourself only as far as you can go and still keep your back straight! Hold 20–30 seconds, change legs.

Tip

If you notice that this stretch causes discomfort in your knee, do exercise 6 instead. You determine the strength of your stretch by leaning more forward or by bringing the leg further in, closer to the chair.

8. Wall Stretch

Starting Position
Find a wall free of obstruction. Lay on your back with one foot against the wall, leg not quite extended. Now, cross the other leg over it.

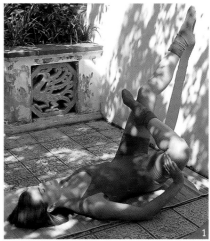

Exercise
Slowly bend the leg that is out-stretched and upright against the wall, sliding your foot down the wall until you feel a stretching of your buttocks muscles. Hold your leg in this position for 20–30 seconds, then change legs.

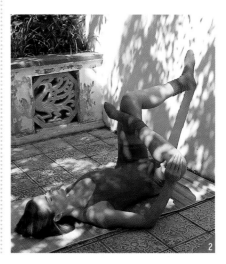

Legs

Strong, Healthy,

Attractive!

Most people are not happy with their legs—they're too short, too fat, too thin. They hate their knees and think that the insides of their thighs are too flabby.

If we work to make them healthy, then our legs will automatically be more attractive!

Exercises for the Legs

Many of my clients are dissatisfied with the appearance of their legs. When they learn that their leg muscles are not functioning as efficiently or harmoniously as they could, they suddenly realize that the underlying muscle tissue must be put in order before the outside can look better!

The muscles that form the fleshy bulk covering the front of the thigh are the quadriceps, a group consisting of four functionally linked muscles, and the sartorius, the longest muscle in the body. This powerful muscle group is responsible for such daily activities as standing, walking, bending down and running and is already strong without special exercise. The quadriceps is made up of the rectus femoris, which runs down the middle of the thigh, the vastus medialis, responsible for the knee's tracking function, and the vastus lateralis and intermedius muscles.

The quadriceps straightens the knee; its antagonist, the hamstrings, lie in the back portion of the leg and are responsible for flexing the knee. This muscle group consists of the semitendinosus and the semimembranosus muscles, which extend down the inner part of the back of the thigh, and a third muscle, the biceps femoris, that lies on the outer side of the thigh. The name "hamstrings" probably relates to the fact that they are relatively inflexible as compared to other major muscle groups. In comparison to the quadriceps group, this muscle group is weaker and tends to be tighter and often short. Generally the ratio of strength in the two muscle groups should be quadriceps to hamstrings 60–40 percent, though some orthopedists claim 70–30 percent is desirable. Although this seems to be a rather unequal ratio, a great number of people suffer from an even greater imbalance of strength. It is very important to stretch the hamstring group daily and to strength-train to balance out the ratio to the above acceptable percentages!

Technique Tips for Exercising the Legs

❶ The knee is one of the more vulnerable joints in our body. Football and soccer players are especially aware of the need for regular strengthening exercises for the muscles around the knee joint. One, the vastus medialus, is of utmost importance to knee stabilization and tracking. Women with broad hips often have knee problems from weak or improper tracking, suffering from knock-knees. This

muscle is optimally trained when you extend your leg fully with a neutral foot. If you have knee problems, extending your knee and tensing your muscles 8–16 times per leg daily will bring improvement.

❷ Pay attention to foot positioning. How you hold your foot during a given exercise determines the effect the exercise will have on the muscle.

❸ Be careful about posture. Keep your back straight if you are sitting or lying, and in neutral position if you are standing. Abdominals are pulled together and tight throughout all the exercises.

❹ When training the hamstrings in a prone position, make sure that your hips remain "glued" to the ground or the bench.

❺ Make every movement count by working in a slow and controlled manner.

❻ Concentrate on your breathing—inhale before you start, exhale on the contraction, and inhale on the release!

1. Seated Leg Extensions (combat knee problems)

Starting Position
Maria's back is straight, arms at sides, abs tight. She wears 2-lb. ankle weights. Her working foot rests on the heel. Her thighs are completely on the bench.

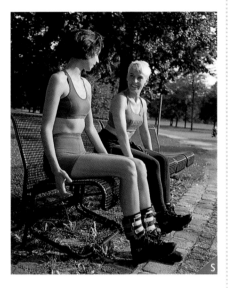

Exercise
Maria fully extends the working leg, then lowers it without actually setting it down on the ground. Throughout the exercise, Maria demonstrates the correct posture for doing the exercise. (My job, in this instance, is to show you how *not* to sit!)

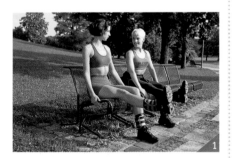

Reps
- 16–32× without weights, 3 sets (or 3× a day)
- 8–24× with ankle weights, 3 sets

2. Three-Way Leg Extension (knee stabilization)

Starting Position
Maria and Amanda, here, are both in position, half lying/half sitting. A rubber band encircles the ankle of the bent leg and the foot of the working leg. They hold their upper bodies up using their forearms, and are careful to keep their shoulders pressed down. The working leg is *slightly* bent to begin with.

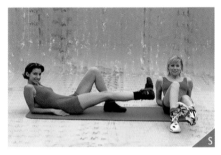

Step 1
Rotate working leg inward so toe points to middle of body, as Amanda demonstrates. Now, pretend you are sitting on a beach and push your heel into the sand—this is how you push the heel to straighten your leg. Hold the tension for a count of 2, then release and relax the knee but don't bend it. The range of motion in this exercise is minimal, but it is very effective if you do it right.

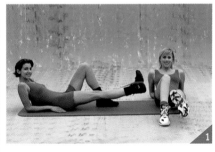

Step 2
Now rotate the leg so that the knee and the toe are pointing to the ceiling. Repeat the extension in step 1 with the foot in this position.

Step 3
Now rotate the leg outward so that the knee and toe are facing away from your body. Extend the leg fully and then release as in the other two steps. This exercise may be done in a chair as well, so perfect at the office!

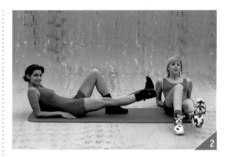

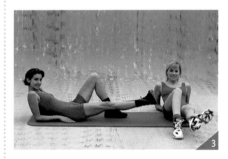

Reps
- Without band, each step 16×; change legs (3× a day)
- With band, each step 8×; change legs (3 sets or 3× a day)

Tip
Think "extend and release"; it's a small movement. The leg must be fully straightened, stretched out, for effectiveness.

3. Leg Extension—Seated on Floor

Starting Position
Wrap a rubber band around the bent leg and the ankle of the working leg and hold the back of the extended working leg just below the knee joint. Lean back, keeping back straight and pulling your abs tight. Your arms and trunk create a natural resistance that stabilizes you and makes the exercise easier to do.

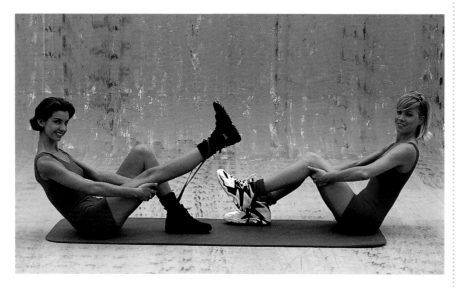

Exercise
Extend your lower leg upward and straighten leg completely. Keep your knees parallel to one another. Slowly lower your leg without putting it on the floor. Make sure to exhale on the extension and inhale as you bring the leg down.

Variation
Wrap the rubber band around the foot of the bent leg instead of just around the leg; it will give you more resistance and make the exercise more difficult.

Reps
⊏━⊐ Without band 8–16×, with band 4–12×; change legs
⊟━⊟ Without band 12–32×; with band 8–16×; change legs

Tip

Remember, even though you are leaning back, you must keep your back very straight.
Execute the exercise slowly and with control.
If you need to take a small "breathing" break, inhale/exhale before extending leg again.

Tip

Remember to pull your abs tight throughout this exercise. It helps you to keep your back straight.

4. Face-to-Face Partner Squats

Starting Position
Either hold hands, or onto a bodybar as Maria and Amanda are doing. With arms extended, they "sit back"—weight on heels. Knees are positioned mid-feet.

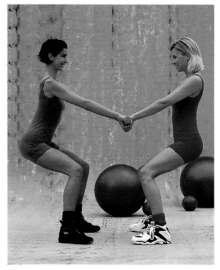

Exercise
Squat down so that the legs form a 90-degree angle. Try to keep your knees over your heels, or no farther than the middle of your feet. When squatting and stretching up, really pull your buttock muscles together.

Reps
⊏━⊐ 4–12×, 2–3 sets
⊟━⊟ 8–16×, 3 sets

Tip

Keep your body neutral at all times. Don't let your chest collapse and your upper back become rounded. If you don't have a partner, do "door squats" (ex. 5, page 94) or hold on to an immovable object! Keep the movements slow and flowing.

5. Double-Duty Partner Squats— Extension and Flexion

Starting Position
Maria, with her legs bent, pushes against Amanda's buttocks. Amanda "sits," her legs bent so knees are over heels. She extends arms for balance.

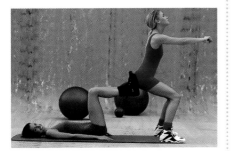

Exercise 1 (static)
Maria pushes with her legs against Amanda, as Amanda pushes against Maria's feet, creating an "isometric" situation. The opposing pushes create tension in their muscle groups, quadriceps and hamstrings, without moving. Hold for 1 minute, 3 sets.

Exercise 2 (dynamic)
Maria positions her legs on Amanda's buttocks and pushes outward, a little forward and upward. Then Amanda pushes backwards, and Maria bends her legs to accommodate the move, but maintains control and tension.

Reps
⌖ 4–8×
⌖ 8–12×

Info
To do this exercise successfully, both partners need balance and control, so work slowly and keep up tension. Remember to change partner positions.

6. Hip-Hop Squats with Bodybar

Starting Position
With bodybar on shoulders, bend legs slightly, just over shoulder-width apart. Body is neutral. Keep the upper back straight, *don't* round shoulders!

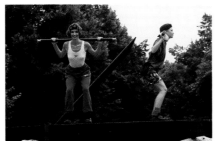

Exercise
Slowly sink down, bringing your buttocks backward, as if to sit. Bring your buttocks no lower than your knees, so that your legs form a 90-degree angle. Slowly rise to return to your starting position.

Reps
⌖ With pole 8–24×
⌖ With bodybar 8–12×, 3 sets

Important
Use a bodybar or weights only after having mastered the squat technique. If you have knee problems, concentrate on ex. 1, 2, 3 before trying squats, and take a wider stance. Also, turn legs and toes slightly outwards, making sure your knees are over your toes.

Tip

Keep upper back erect throughout. Don't lower your buttocks below your knees.

7. Front Lunges

Starting Position
Amanda is in neutral position, standing with legs and feet parallel and a shoulder-width apart. The bodybar is placed on shoulder, as in exercise 6.

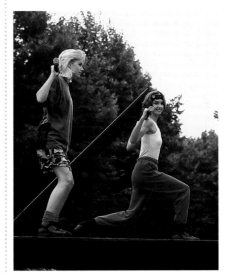

Exercise
Maria, striding forward, softlands on her heel to roll onto the foot. She lowers back leg slightly, her weight over the heel of the lead leg. She maintains a neutral spine, tenses buttocks and abs, then pushes from the heel and returns her lead leg to the start position.

Reps
⌖ With pole 4–8× each leg, or alternate legs, 2 sets
⌖ With bodybar 8–12× each leg, or alternate legs 8–16×, 3 sets

Tip

Keep trunk very stable. Never allow knee to bend over and beyond your toes. Keep the lead leg at a 90-degree angle.

8. Squat Lift Combo

Starting Position
Stand with legs just over shoulder-width apart. With bodybar or pole in front as support, lower yourself to squat position.

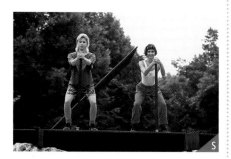

Exercise
Rise up from squat, lifting a leg to the side (do not throw or kick it up). Lower it, going directly back into precise squat position. Now, rise up again, lifting other leg. It's lift, squat, lift, squat. Keep leg straight on lift.

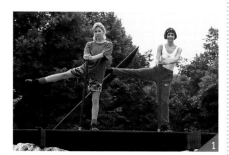

Reps
🔲 4–8×, alternate right/left = 1
🔲 8–16×, overload with reps to one side, then change

Info

Lifting with the knee facing front will work hips and outside leg extensively. Lifting and rotating leg, so knee is facing up, will bring quadriceps more into play.

9. Standing Quadriceps Stretch

Starting Position
Stand on one leg, keeping it slightly bent. Hold other leg by the front of the foot or ankle with your arm flexed. Use your other hand for balance.

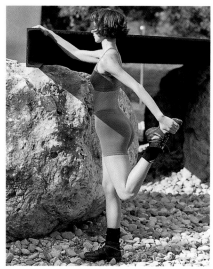

Exercise
Pull your leg farther back and upwards, pushing your hip forward at the same time. This way you create an optimal stretch. Pull your left shoulder forward, but keep your left elbow bent. Hold 20–30 seconds, change legs, 3 sets.

Tip

When pulling your leg back, keep your pelvis facing front at all times. Hold your back straight, shoulders down and abs pulled together!

10. Side-Lying Quadriceps Stretch

Starting Position
Lie on your side, floor leg bent 90 degrees and slightly in front. Grasping the other leg by the ankle, bring it towards the chest.

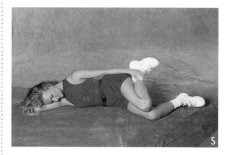

Exercise
Without raising leg, pull the top leg back and push hip and shoulder forward. The elbow is slightly bent. Hold 20–30 seconds, change legs, 3 sets.

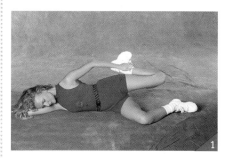

Tip

Keep your body weight slightly forward throughout the stretch. Continue to pull leg back and really push forward with the hip. This creates an optimal stretch in the thigh from the hip flexor to the knee. Remember to keep your hips facing forward; don't roll back into the stretch.

11. Deep Lunge Hip Flexor Stretch

12. Standing Hamstring Curl

Starting Position

Front knee must be over/behind heel and back leg placed so hands can be used as support. Keep back straight, or wait until you're flexible enough.

Starting Position

Standing on your right leg, stretch the left one directly back, so the toes are just touching the floor (no weight on them, please!). Stand close enough to the object you are holding so that your body will remain in a neutral position. Your standing leg is slightly bent but tensed. Your abs are pulled tight.

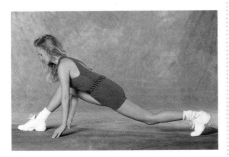

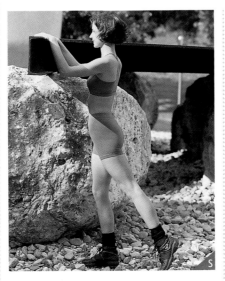 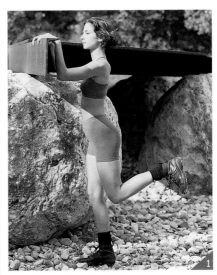

Exercise

Bend the knee of your back leg slightly, until you feel a pulling sensation in the front of your hip (that's your hip flexor saying hello!). Some of you may feel the stretch more in the quadriceps —that's good, too. If you want more stretch in the hip flexor, though, push the hip more forward and bend the back knee more. Your back and head form a diagonal line with your back leg. Abs are pulled tight.

Exercise

Slowly pull lower left leg upwards, keeping the knee in its fixed position. When you feel the muscle in your back thigh tense up, pull your buttocks together and really squeeze the working leg inwards toward the thigh. Slowly lower but don't place toes on the floor.

Reps

- 8-16×, 4-8× with ankle weights; change legs
- 12–20×, 8–16× with ankle weights or bands; change legs

Important

Don't fall into a swayback.

Tip

Both feet must point forward; don't allow back foot to turn to outside.
Also, keep back straight. This is an advanced stretch; if you find yourself "hunching up," wait until you have more flexibility before attempting it.

Info

Overload by using ankle weights, tubing or rubber bands.
Bands: Place band under right foot and around left ankle. Tubing: Make a loop and place around left ankle. Step on tubing with right foot to anchor, and hold remaining tubing.
Keep tension in tubing and rubber band at all times.
Keep movement slow and controlled.

Tip

Keep head, trunk, and upper body stable. Don't rock forward as you pull your back leg up. Shoulders are depressed.

Important

Keep the knee fixed. Just move the lower leg, so you will get an optimal workout in the hamstring muscle.

13. Prone Hamstring Curl on an Inclined Platform

Starting Position

On 3/1 inclined platform, lie with legs stretched out, buttocks pulled together, toes touching floor. Neck and head are extension of back.

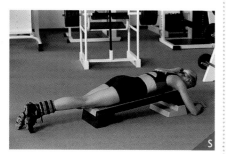

Exercise

Using ankle weights, Loren slowly curls one leg up and in, squeezing buttocks together, then lowers back to start.

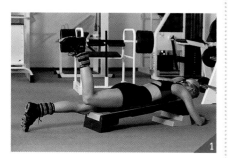

Reps

⊏━⊐ 8–16×; with weights, 4–8×
⊏═⊐ 12–20×; with weights, 8–16×

Tip

Rubber bands can also be used, attach as in exercise 12.
To increase intensity, raise knee of working leg a few inches above platform and do curls while holding it in position, steady throughout. Keep pelvis directly on the platform.

14. Supine Hip Lift

Starting Position

Start in supine position, bent legs shoulder-width apart, feet flexed, weight in your heels. Daniela has taken a broom handle and placed it across her hips as a reminder to keep the pelvis down. Her head is resting comfortably, her shoulders are depressed and her neck is long.

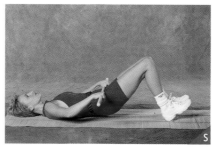

Your extended leg is the weight, so keep it at the same height throughout exercise. Now raise your buttocks and, as before, hold and squeeze. Really use supporting leg to do the work, and keep the extended leg steady.

Reps

⊏━⊐ With pole, 8–12×; bodybar, 4-8×
⊏═⊐ With pole, 12–20×; bodybar, 8–16×; with a leg extended, 8–12×

Exercise

Push buttocks upwards until tension builds in hamstrings. At top of the lift, hold and squeeze buttocks and tense hamstrings 10–20 seconds. Leave at least ¾ of your back on the floor and really dig in with your heels.

Variation

⊏═⊐ For advanced exercisers only, from position above, place one foot flat on floor and extend the other leg hip height, absolutely parallel to floor.

Tip

Place support leg far enough from buttocks to really work hamstring. If leg is too close, you work buttocks more than legs. Important! Keep most of your back on the floor. Don't lift onto shoulder blades or neck! Keep lifted leg low.

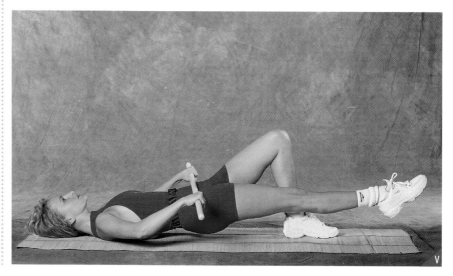

15. Double-Duty Hamstring Curl with Partner Rowing

Starting Position
On 1/3 platform, Amanda lies with head and neck aligned with spine. Her knees are *on* the platform, tubing taut around shins. Maria sits straight.

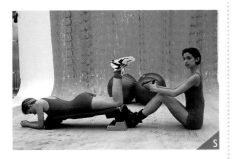

Exercise
Squeezing buttocks together, Amanda presses hips into platform and pulls legs toward her buttocks. At the same time, Maria, back straight, pulls her arms back, providing even more tension in the already taut tubing.

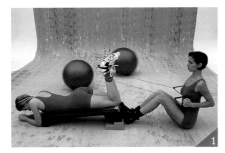

Reps
 4–12×; change partner positions
8–16×;change partner positions

Tip

Create a good rhythm with your partner, tubing pulled and legs curled simultaneously.
Make sure the hips press into the platform as the legs are pulled back.

16. Prone Hamstring Stretch with Partner

Starting Position
Lie back, in relaxed position, with legs outstretched. Tighten abs. Shoulders are depressed, neck is long. Okay to put something under neck to cushion.

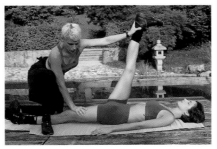

Exercise
Kneeling, partner helps to raise leg. It must be kept straight; lift only as high as leg stays straight. Press gently on thigh of outstretched leg to help stretch hip flexors. Slowly and carefully, gently push upstretched leg toward partner, who directs amount of pressure. First, partner takes deep breath. On exhale, the leg is gently pushed a bit farther. Hold each position, inhale–exhale, then repeat.

Variation
If partnerless, place towel around lower leg and pull it upward towards you. Repeat, breathing as above. Keep head flat during stretch. If advanced, and you can, hold your leg with your hands. Be gentle and graduate range of motion slowly. Hold each stretch 20–30 seconds. Change legs.

Tip

Keep head and buttocks on floor.
If leg starts to quiver from tension, shake it out and start again

17. Standing Hamstring Stretch

Starting Position
Supporting leg is flexed, toes and knee point forward. Place leg to be stretched at a height on a chair or stoop that allows the back to be kept straight.

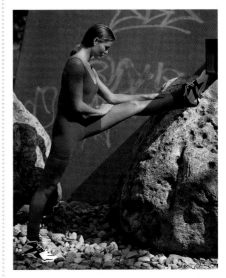

Exercise
Slowly bend over towards your outstretched leg, keeping your abs tight and your back absolutely straight. As soon as you feel a pulling sensation in the back of your leg, stop, take a deep breath, and then gently move a little lower, exhaling as you go. Hold 20–30 seconds each stretch phase. Change legs.

Tip

Pull your shoulder blades together and push your chest out as you bend over. Remember to place the leg low if you are not very flexible.

Adductors and Abductors

The adductor muscles are rightly classified under "legs," whereas the abductors are actually part of the "buttocks." As the abductors, however, are antagonists to the adductors, they are best covered together—here in this special leg exercise section.

About 90% of my female clients first come to me because of the flab or fat that they have, or imagine they have, on their hips and inner thighs. Those suffering from cellulite or who always tend to gain weight in those body areas have, more often than not, inherited those genes. These exercises will not magically melt the fat from those areas, but they will firm up and activate the muscle fibers there which will, in turn, help to give you better form and definition. If the muscles are healthy, the blood flows more freely, and circulation is better. Thus, the chance for burning fat in those hard-to-get-at areas will increase when you train cardiovascularly.

When you lift your leg away from you, the abductor muscles are doing their work. These muscles lie behind your hip and are made up of two main muscles, gluteus medius and the smaller gluteus minimus, both lying above and to the side of the gluteus maximus that forms the somewhat fleshy part of your buttock. The abductor group is also supported in its function by six little muscles of the hip rotator group which lies under the gluteal muscles. When you see a Lower-Body Workout group fitness class, you will undoubtedly see thousands of abductor exercises within 60 minutes! Really important, however, is the job the abductors perform by stabilizing your pelvis.

The antagonist to the abductor is, of course, the adductor group which pulls the leg inwards toward the body. This muscle group on the inner side of the thigh consists of five muscles: adductor magnus, adductor longus, adductor brevis, pectineus, and gracilis. You notice how weak these muscles are if you have ever ridden a horse, or done in-line or ice skating. They also help to stabilize, but tend to be very inflexible, especially because we sit so very much. So we need to stretch, stretch and stretch again this muscle group.

Technique Tips for Working the Adductor/Abductor Muscles

❶ **Exercises for these muscle groups can be done either standing or in a recline position. Standing, you are passively working the supporting leg as well, because it must stabilize the body. Be sure to keep your body neutral throughout the exercise.**
❷ **If you exercise while lying on your side, you will be better able to isolate the working muscle. You are also working against gravity as well.**
❸ **When working on your side, hold your position steady. Don't fall forward or backward!**
❹ **Don't forget your breathing technique. Inhale as you start the exercise, exhale during contraction.**
❺ **Keep a neutral foot when working a leg; hold the foot in a stable, but not contracted, position. This lets the energy flow better to the working muscle.**
❻ **If your body type tends to build little mountains on the sides of your hips, don't overdo the abductor exercises. However, exercises for both adductors and abductors are not just for cosmetic reasons. These muscles serve a very important stabilizing function. Include them in your training at least once a week.**
❼ **When performing adductor exercises while in a side-lying position, make sure that your hips are aligned one directly over the other; I call it "stacking" the hips.**

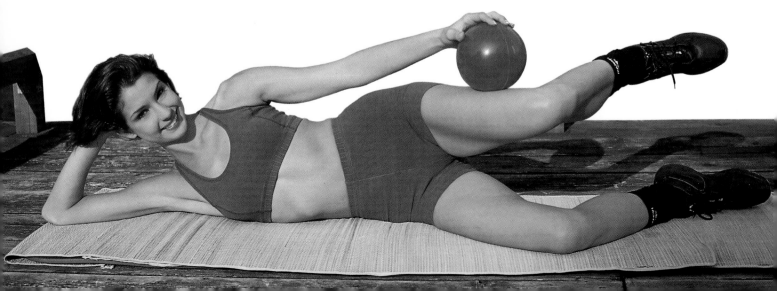

18. Standing Abductor/Adductor Exercises with Tubing

Starting Position
Debbie has looped one end of the tubing around a tree and the other around her foot. To make a loop, take the tubing handle and pull the other end through it. Debbie stands near the tree for good body alignment, her legs about hip-width apart, the supporting leg slightly bent. Her hand is against the tree for balance.

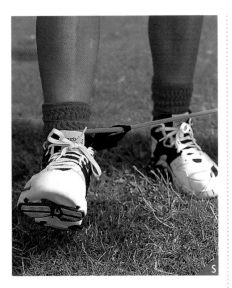

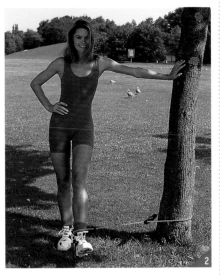

Step 1: Abductors
Debbie has tubing, under tension, looped around her outside lower leg. Slowly, she lifts her leg outwards and away from her, always keeping her

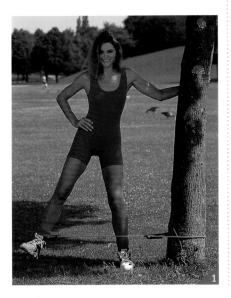

knee facing forward. Her foot is in a stable and neutral position.

Step 2: Adductors
Debbie, tubing looped around her inside leg, pulls this working leg inward, and across her front. She directs the movement with her heel.

Reps
 4–12×; change sides and legs
8–24×; change sides and legs

Tip
Keep working leg straight and the tubing under constant tension. Watch your posture. Don't lean into the movement. Stand straight, maintaining a neutral position throughout the exercise.

19. Side-Lying Adductor Training with Platform

Starting Position
Loren lies beside platform, one leg bent, one extended. Her aligned hips determine distance. Arms are placed for comfort. Head down relaxes spine.

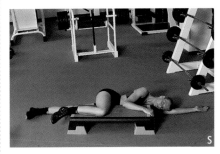

Exercise
Slowly, Loren raises floor leg towards ceiling, keeping a neutral foot and straight leg on the lift. She lowers leg, but not to the floor.

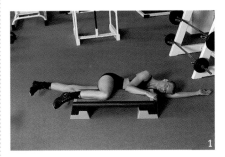

Reps
4–12×; change legs
8–24×; change legs

Tip

Keep your abs tight throughout the workout. Make sure your hips are correctly positioned, stacked one on top of the other.

20. Side-Lying Abductor/Adductor Exercises with Ball

Starting Position
Lie on your side with your legs bent, knees slightly forward and lower legs behind. Your heels should be in line with your buttocks. Maintain this position throughout the exercise. It will help you to avoid falling backwards, which is a common mistake.

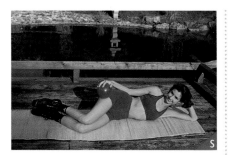

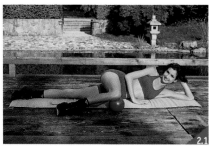

Step 1: Abductors
Place a ball, or a grapefruit or something else that will roll and has some weight to it, on your upper thigh. Now, raise your upper leg, keeping the legs parallel to one another. (Do not rotate the working leg backwards!) As you lift the leg, roll the ball down the side of your thigh in the direction of your knee. Pull the buttock muscles together and slowly bring the leg back down, rolling the ball back up to the hip. Keep a neutral foot throughout the exercise.

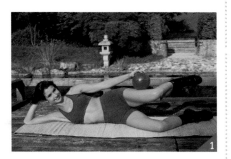

Step 2: Adductors
Place a ball under the knee of the top bent leg. This will provide balance. Extend the floor leg, keeping the hips stacked over one another.

Now, slowly raise the floor leg, as was done in exercise 19. Lower the leg, but without putting it on the floor.

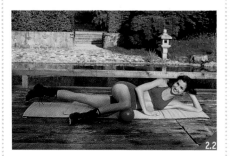

Reps
🏋 4–12×; change legs
🏋 8–24×; change legs

Tip
It's best to lie flat, as in exercise 19, so your spine remains neutral and relaxed—but Maria likes posing! Don't forget your breathing technique. Squeeze the buttock muscles together when working the floor leg.

21. Supine Wall Adductor Stretch

Starting Position
Find wall space—move furniture! Lie down and "skooch" buttocks up to wall. Walk legs up, keeping back and head relaxed, arms out to sides.

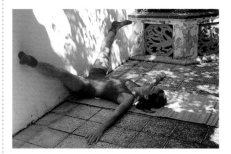

Exercise
Open legs wide enough to feel a pull in the inner thighs. This exercise, with the legs supported, is easy on the back. Hold 20–30 seconds in each phase.

Variation 1
If wall space is scarce, lie on back, head relaxed on floor, and bend legs, bringing them to your chest. Holding your ankles, open your legs outwards in bent position. For more resistance, push elbows into the inside of your knees, pushing legs out farther. The experienced and flexible may extend legs for a more intense stretch.

Variation 2
This standard is very advanced and not for everybody. Sit on the floor and spread your legs outwards. Keep trunk and head very straight, arms extended, fingertips touching the floor. Now lean forward to feel pull in the inner thighs.

Tip
Try to really *relax* into these stretches.

22. Side-Lying Abductor Stretch

Starting Position
Lie in a supine position, both legs extended. Keep your neck long and let your arms rest by your side. Bend left leg and pull it up towards your body.

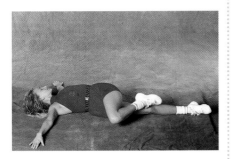

Stretch
Place your right hand on the outside of your left knee and push the leg downward across your body, as Daniela has done, then stretch both arms out in line with shoulders. Both shoulder blades must be touching the floor. Hold 20–30 seconds and change sides.

Tip

Adjust knee for a pulling sensation in hip, obliques, and chest.
For more hip stretch, use the hand opposite the crossed leg. Push knee towards floor, holding pressure to increase stretch intensity.
If you do this, be sure head, neck, and both shoulder blades remain on the floor.

Important

If you have spine problems, *don't push* the knee down. Exercise moderately. If you have ever had a slipped disc, avoid this exercise unless otherwise recommended by your physical therapist.

23. Pretzel Stretch—Seated Abductor Stretch

Starting Position
Start in position seated on floor, legs extended out in front. Now cross left leg over the right. Extended leg will be bent towards your body.

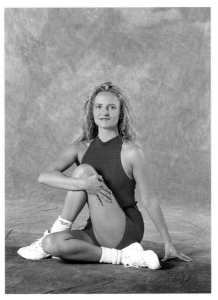

Exercise
Cradle your right arm around your left leg, as Daniela is demonstrating. Now, pull the leg towards your chest and turn your upper body slightly into the crossed leg. Your back stays absolutely straight and your left arm is extended. Shoulders are depressed. Hold 20–30 seconds. Change sides.

Tip

If the position in the photo is too hard for you to execute, leave the right leg extended.
Remember that for a really effective stretch, both buttocks should be on the floor at all times.

24. Half Moon Stretch— Standing Abductor Stretch

Starting Position
Cross your right leg over your left. Press the feet together and bend your legs slightly. You maintain a neutral posture throughout the stretch.

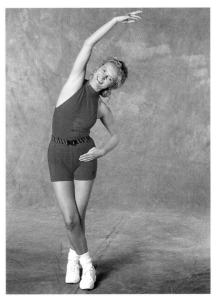

Exercise
Extend your right arm to the side and overhead. Your left arm works as a support by holding your hip, as Daniela demonstrates. Remember to keep your shoulders down. Now push your right hip slightly outward to increase the intensity of the stretch. Hold 20–30 seconds. Change legs.

Tip

Really bend to the side.
Don't lean your upper body either forward or backward!
(See ex. 15 for upper backs.)

The Calves

Improve Form

and Function

Are your calves the bane of your life? Too thin or too hefty? Your calves are often the forgotten muscle in your exercise plan. Exercising them will not make them enormous—quite the contrary. Definition and strength are what we are striving for.

Exercises for the Calves

Surely you've noticed the appearance of calf muscles in people who wear high heels—yes, even some men wear higher heels! The calf definition is clear. This should say something about what raising and lowering shoe or boot heel height can achieve for the calf muscles. However, if you enjoy wearing high heels much of the time, you run the risk of a very shortened Achilles tendon, which can lead to injuries or chronic discomfort. It's important for many of us to spend more time stretching our calf muscles!

The calf muscles reside in the lower leg. The gastrocnemius and soleus form the main bulk of the calf musculature. The gastrocnemius forms the bulky part of your calf, and extends from just above the back of the knee to your heel. The soleus lies under the gastrocnemius, originating at the back of your leg bones (tibia and fibula) and running into the Achilles tendon, which attaches to your heel. Both these muscles contract to pull your heel back and up, when you point your toes down or stand on your toes. They create resilience when you walk, run, jump or hop. The gastrocnemius plays a role in helping to bend your knee, especially if the hamstrings are weak. The soleus doesn't affect the knee; it primarily flexes the foot downward.

Techniques and Tips for Exercising Your Calves

❶ Because of how the muscle is attached, you train the soleus more effectively when your knees are bent. If you think your calves are too thin, concentrate on exercising this muscle a little more often.

❷ When your leg is straight, you can train your gastrocnemius muscle more effectively. If you are unhappy with your calves, they look "stumpy" or are too thick, concentrate on training this muscle more often than the soleus. With the correct amount of exercise, you can create definition in your lower leg and activate the muscle fibers so that fat within the muscle fiber has a better chance of being burned off when you are exercising cardiovascularly.

❸ As with all the other exercises, train prudently. Don't start off doing more than you can really handle. Perform each of the training and stretching exercises *slowly*, concentrating on the feel of the muscles as they work, keeping movements under good control.

❹ When raising your heel, really raise it to the full height. Working the "full range of motion" is paramount to success.

❺ When performing standing heel raises for the gastrocnemius, be sure your working leg is *completely* straight while lifting and lowering the heel. The body moves up and down, *not forward and back*.

❻ Remember your breathing technique. Inhale at the start of the exercise, exhale during!

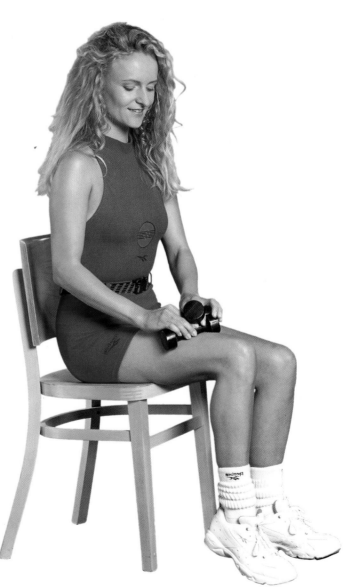

1. Standing Heel Raise in Back-Lunge Position

Starting Position

Daniela is standing in a lunge position. Her front leg is bent, knee slightly behind her heel. Her back leg is extended and her heel is flat on the floor. Both feet are facing forward; her trunk and hips are also facing forward. Chest is high and shoulders depressed.

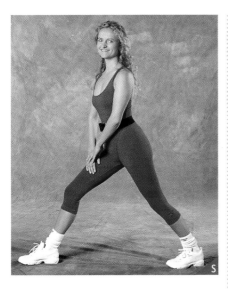

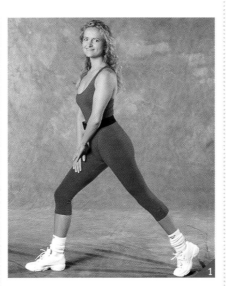

Exercise

Daniela lifts her heel until her weight is on the ball of her foot. She raises it as high as she can, feeling the gastrocnemius tighten, then lowers it slowly.

Reps

8–12×; change legs
12–24×; change legs

Tip

If, in the beginning, you find the number of reps too much for you, do only what you can.
Many people have an amazing amount of tension in the calf muscles and tend to cramp easily; if so, stretch between sets and take a little longer before resuming your reps.
Be sure you come up only to the ball of your foot, *not* onto your toes. You must feel the weight in the ball of your foot, or you are doing the exercise improperly.

Tip

Keep the upper body very still, chest out and shoulders down and back.
The movement in this exercise is vertical, up and down, *not* forward and back.
Make sure you really put the foot through its full range of motion.
Execute your movement slowly.

2. Standing Heel Raise in Back-Lunge Position —Flexed

Starting Position

Daniela's stance here is somewhat like the one in exercise 1, except that here her back leg is bent.

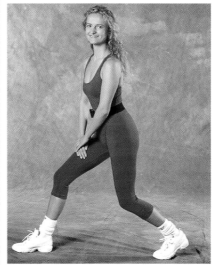

Exercise

In this bent knee position, raise and lower your heel, slowly. Keep the back knee bent throughout the exercise.

Reps

8–12×; change legs
12–24×; change legs

Tip

Make sure that just the back foot moves.
The upper body is held straight and still.
Keep your hips facing forward.
Come up only to the ball of your foot, *not* your toes.
Done properly, you must feel the weight in the ball of your foot.

3. Standing Heel Raise with Hand Weights

4. Standing Heel Raise with Hand Weights—Flexed

Starting Position

Stand with your legs placed hip-width apart. Hold the weights on your shoulders, with bent arms, elbows out, and shoulders down.

Starting Position

Stand with your legs bent and placed confortably hip-width apart. Hold the weights on your shoulders with arms bent, elbows out, shoulders depressed. Really remember to tighten your abs. This will help you to maintain your balance during the exercise.

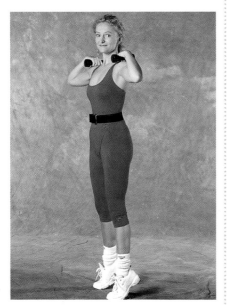

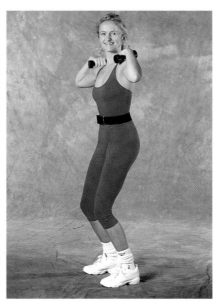

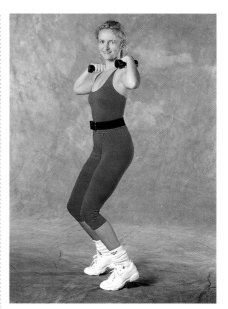

Exercise

Keeping the legs very straight, raise up on to the balls of your feet. Squeeze your buttock muscles together and pull the abs together; this will help you keep your balance. Slowly lower the heels to the floor.

Exercise

In this bent knee position, raise up to the balls of your feet. This is not easy because of the balance problem. So concentrate. Build a nice steady rhythm—not too fast.

Reps

⊂━⊃ 4–8×
⊊━⊋ 8–16×

Reps

⊂━⊃ 4–8×
⊊━⊋ 8–16×

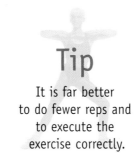

Tip

This exercise demands a lot of concentration in order to keep your balance and maintain technique. Make sure you are coming up onto the balls of your feet, and *not* onto your toes!

Tip

It is far better to do fewer reps and to execute the exercise correctly.

Info

If you have trouble with balance or tend to have muscle cramps, perform this exercise without using hand weights. Place your hands on your hips instead. If you can hold onto something for balance, by all means do so, just remember to keep your posture correct. If you have knee problems, I recommend that you do soleus exercises in a seated position.

5. Standing Combo Heel Raise with Pole

Starting Position

Take a *plié* stance, legs wide enough to keep the knees over the heels, but allowing a free range of motion in the foot. Hold the pole vertically out in front of you so that you can maintain a neutral position, shoulders down, neck long and head straight. Hold the pole with both hands, keeping the arms relaxed. This two-joint exercise is very effective—if it is *executed properly!*

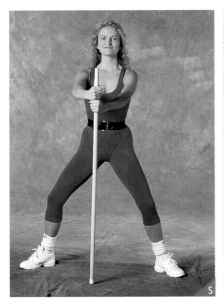

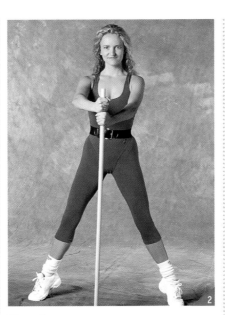

Step 1
With knees still bent, raise your heels.

Step 2
Straighten legs with heels still raised.

Step 3
With heels still raised, bend legs again.

Step 4
In the bent position, lower your heels.

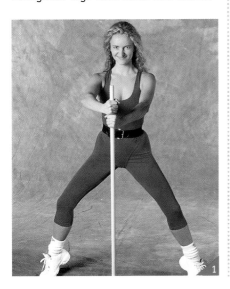

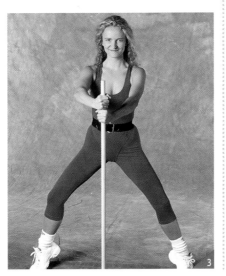

Variation

Starting position as in exercise 3 (legs hip-width and straight).

Step 1 Raise heels with straight legs.

Step 2 Still on the balls of your feet, bend your knees.

Step 3 Still on the balls of your feet, straighten legs again.

Step 4 Lower your heels to start.

Reps

The complete combo

4–12×

8–24×

Info

This exercise combination is one of the most demanding, coordinationwise, of all those in the book. If you don't understand it or cannot perform it comfortably, leave it for later.
If you do want to try it, just reduce the number of repetitions and do more sets!

Tip

Remember to keep a neutral position. Watch how and where you hold the pole.
Don't open your legs too wide, or you will have trouble raising your heels. Find a comfortable stance that allows full range of motion and good technique.

6. Standing One-Leg Heel Raise

Starting Position
Place a foot on a raised object; Daniela uses phone books. The slightly bent knee of the supporting leg must be over the heel or middle foot, *not* over the toes. Place your hands behind the back, elbows pointing slightly back. Keep chest high and body neutral. Start with foot of working leg flat on floor. Pull abs together!

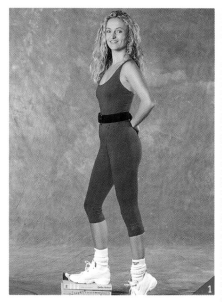
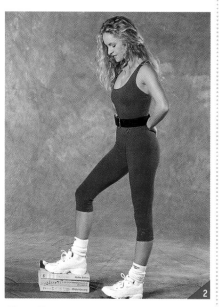

Step 1
Raise up on to the ball of your foot, keeping a straight working leg. The supporting leg and foot remain stable and without movement. Make sure your movement is vertical, i.e., up and down, when you raise your heel.

Step 2
When lowering your heel, you can roll back on to it, lifting the toes slightly. In this way, you will automatically slightly stretch the calf muscle, creating a true range of motion.

Reps
⬤━⬤ 4–12×; change legs
⬤━⬤ 8–24×; change legs

Important
Make sure that the knee of the supporting leg is kept bent throughout the exercise.
It is also important to keep the knee positioned over the heel or mid-foot to avoid pressure to the knee joint.

Tip
Remember to keep a neutral position throughout.
Pull the elbows back; this will help to lift your chest.
Make sure not to fall into a swayback.
Keep the shoulders down.

7. Seated Heel Raise with Hand Weights (for the soleus)

Starting Position
Sit with the legs at a 90-degree angle and feet flat on the floor. Keeping the back straight, place the weights on your thighs, *not* on the knees!

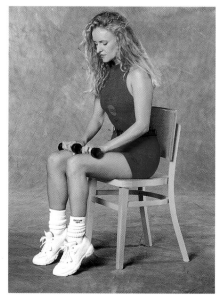

Exercise
Raise both heels while pressing down with the weights. Slowly lower.

Reps
⬤━⬤ (1 leg) 4–12×; change legs
(2 legs) 4–12×
⬤━⬤ (1 leg) 8–24×; change legs
(2 legs) 8–24×

Variation
4–12× right leg, 4–12× both legs, 4–12× left leg, 4–12× both legs, then alternate right and left 4–12×

Tip
Sit straight; keep weights mid-thigh. Roll up only to balls of feet, *not* onto toes. Keep knees in place, don't let them wobble around.

8. Standing Heel Raises on Riser with Pole

Starting Position
Stand on something that will allow you to lower your heels without hitting the floor, or it tipping over! Daniela uses a pole for balance, to concentrate on the full range of motion in her feet. Place your feet so you can comfortably raise up onto the balls. Your heels are slightly lowered. Posture correct—need I say more?

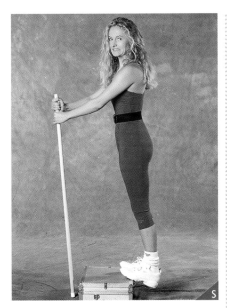
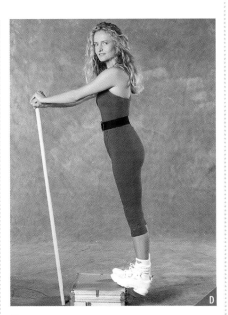

Exercise
Raise up as high as you can on to the balls of your feet (1 below). Slowly lower heels back to start position.

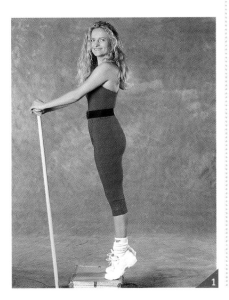

Reps
4–12×
8–24×

Double-Duty
Use the down side of the exercise as a stretch (see D above). Lower heels as far as they can go and hold for 20–30 seconds. Repeat at least three times!

Tip
Take care to choose a stable object to stand on. If you hold onto something, position it at a distance that will allow you to maintain good alignment and posture.

9. Standing Calf Stretch in Back Lunge Position

Starting Position
Lunge position: front leg bent, knee behind heel; back leg extended, heel flat. Feet, trunk, and hips face forward. You feel pulling in calf.

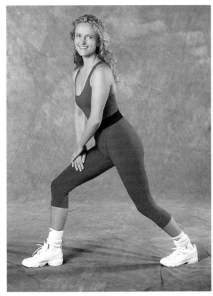

Exercise
First extend back of leg fully and feel the pull in the large calf muscle. Now bend your knee, keeping the heel on the floor. You should feel the stretch transfer to the lower part of the calf. Keep the knee bent and the heel flat on the floor. Hold 30 seconds. Change legs, repeat several times.

Tip
Keep the whole body in correct alignment: chest high, shoulders back and down. Your body should build a diagonal line from head to foot. If your knee hurts when stretching the soleus, do exercise 8 stretch with bent knees.

V. Aerobics? let's Call It Cardiovascular Training

When aerobic training is mentioned, many people think of Jane Fonda. Today, aerobics is specific training for the cardiovascular (CV) system or the cardiorespiratory system.

Cardio comes from the Greek word "*kardia*," for heart. In today's vernacular, it refers to our heart and its function of pumping blood through our vast system of blood vessels. "Respiratory" refers to our lungs and their function of taking in oxygen, within their own walls and those of our cells, and expelling carbon dioxide. Your cardiovascular system is the key factor in the performance of any sport requiring more than a few minutes of sustained activity. For every movement, our muscles use energy to carry out the activity. The energy for muscle contraction is supplied by an enzyme called adenosinetriphosphat, ATP for short, which each muscle has in limited quantity. This energy reserve aids the muscle for only about ten seconds; after that it is depleted and must be replenished. There are several methods that our body uses to accomplish this.

Aerobic System

"Aerobic" means "with oxygen." In this system, fatty acids and glucose (carbohydrates) are broken down in the presence of oxygen. The stored body fat is released into the bloodstream and sent to the muscles as fuel to produce energy. Fat can be burned only in the presence of oxygen, and the by-products, carbon dioxide and water, that are produced from this process don't lead to early muscle fatigue, as does the by-product lactic acid in the anaerobic system.

Anaerobic System

The anaerobic system uses glucose too, but it does not burn fatty acids. It relies on immediate energy stores (the phosphagen system, or ATP-CP) and short-term energy (lactic acid) systems. If the exercise is very intense and of short duration, such as a 100-yard dash, resistance training or running for a bus, you are using ATP and CP, immediate and short-term anaerobic energy systems.

When we are at rest, our muscles are aerobic. Actually, under normal circumstances, our bodies are always aerobic. Our heart, brain, and nerves all need oxygen to function, so *we* are aerobic

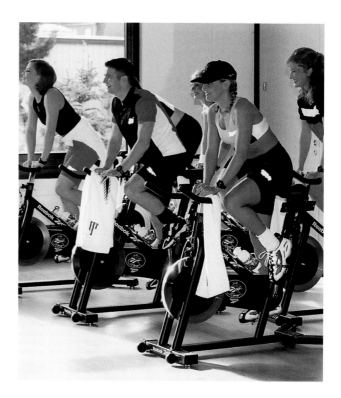

Aerobic:
Fat and carbohydrates are broken down in the presence of oxygen to produce energy. Water and carbon dioxide are the by-products. When we work aerobically, we can exercise longer and burn fat efficiently.

Anaerobic:
Carbohydrates and the intramuscularly-stored ATP-CP reserves are called upon to help us perform intense, short-term activities. The by-product of this process is lactic acid.

beings! This means that all our normal daily activities, like walking, washing the car, vacuum cleaning, or taking out the trash and recyclables, are aerobic. What happens, though, when you walk up the stairs? Do you get out of breath right away? Well, this is when the muscles start to work anaerobically!

Muscle Soreness

After you exercise, there are three different kinds of muscle soreness you could experience. The first is that "burn" during exercise, or immediately after intense exercise, during the cool-down phase. This type of soreness is usually transitory and is related to lactic acid build-up during the anaerobic phase of your training. Lactic acid clears from the body in about 30-60 minutes.

Soreness and stiffness that you experience in your muscles one to days later is referred to as delayed-onset muscle soreness (DOMS) and is an indication that the body is adapting to the demands of exercise with which it is not familiar. Muscle soreness can occur because you have just started an exercise program and your body is unaccustomed to the demand. It can occur in well-trained exercisers who have taken a break and are resuming their activities. Even if you are a toughie, every time you change intensity, duration, or frequency your body will most likely signal your progression with DOMS.

The pain that you experience is caused by tiny micro-traumas in the muscle fibers that have occurred during a specific exercise or training movement. About one to two hours after your workout, white blood cells build up in the affected area in order to eliminate dead cells. This process always causes the muscle cells to regenerate. Fluid usually gathers in the tiny tears, causing slight swelling and making the muscle tight or sore. This swelling is not usually detectable by the human eye. But it is certainly felt. There are only theories as to why DOMS occurs so late and not immediately after exercise. European researchers feel that it has to do with the absence of nerve receptors in the affected muscle fibers. There are only a few receptors on the outside of the muscle cells and they obviously take longer to transmit the message to the brain. Therefore, we get the news about our soreness only much later.

Not so long ago—and to some even today—muscle soreness was seen as guaranteeing a really good workout. Today, we think differently. A well-constructed workout will help avoid muscle soreness. If you are a beginner, or returning to training after an absence, it's best to keep the intensity and resistance low and build up slowly. Even if you consider yourself a toughie, change only one program element, not everything at once. Good ways to reduce or avoid muscle soreness are to take the time to warm-up properly, choose appropriate movements, and include enough time in your workout for post-exercise stretching. Remember, if you want to strengthen, you must stretch as well!

Why do we experience post-exercise muscle soreness one or two days after exercise? The exact cause of this phenomena is not certain. McArdle et al., 1991, believe it has to do with negative or eccentric muscular contractions. European research tells us that the muscle fibers are

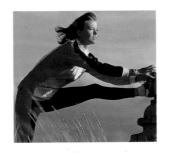

outside of the cells take longer to transmit the message of muscle soreness to the brain, hence

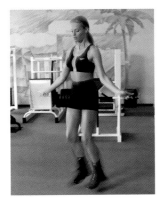

not equipped with receptors that can immediately transmit the messages to the brain. The few receptors on the

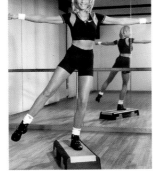

the delayed reaction of 24 to 48 hours. Usually, muscle soreness disappears after about three or four days.

Important: If stretching and other daily activities are causing you pain in an exercised body part, you might have had a muscle strain or tear. If this is likely, check with your doctor immediately!

Lactic Acid

Many exercises associate lactic acid with DOMS. Actually this is not the case. Lactic acid is a natural by-product of the anaerobic effort and, when sufficient oxygen becomes available, it can be metabolized and used for energy. Lactate is the "salt" of the lactic acid. Lactate blocks the metabolism of fat. If too much lactic acid accumulates in the muscle, it becomes so fatigued that it can no longer carry on.

Most people in our fitness centers are interested in cardiovascular or aerobic training because it burns fat more efficiently. If those exercisers choose an aerobic activity like walking, jogging or biking and maintain a training heart rate between 50–75% of their maximum, they will be "working with oxygen." At one time it was said that you had to exercise for at least 30 minutes before you would start burning fat. This has been overruled by the experts. As I mentioned before, even at rest we are in a constant state of oxygenation; this means that so long as we don't undertake an activity that makes us "anaerobic," we will still be burning fat, because fat is burned in the presence of oxygen. This means that even a 10-minute walk will help activate your cardiovascular system. This is, of course, not to say that it isn't better to exercise longer. It certainly is a more efficient way to train, and you will see results in a shorter time. But *every* movement counts. Better less, than nothing at all!

As soon as you reach a peak in your cardiovascular exercise where you go from working with oxygen to becoming anaerobic, where you have a significant increase in breathing, your muscles start burning and you have the feeling you need to slow your pace, you have arrived at your *anaerobic threshold.*

We all know how important our heart muscle is. Few of us consciously think about training it as a muscle. Most exercisers just want to burn fat. It is important to train the heart in different ways just as we do our other bodily muscles. We can train in a *steady state;* that means keeping our heart rate between 50–75% of our maximum. If you have been training longer and want to train for cardiovascular condition, you will train above 75%.

The best way to train in order to raise your anaerobic threshold is "interval fitness" training. This type of training will not burn fat as efficiently, because you will be working anaerobically for short periods, but it is essential for raising your anaerobic threshold and is a tool in training your heart to work more efficiently. With this type of training, I can help my clients lower their resting heart rates over time. A lower resting heart rate means that your heart doesn't have to beat as often, but delivers as much or more blood to the body. This is economy!

Effects of Cardiovascular Training

Physiological

- Higher metabolic rate—more calories burned at rest
- Prevention of cardiovascular diseases, such as arteriosclerosis and hypertension
- Improves ability of heart to pump blood (stroke volume), oxygen consumption (VO2 max), and motor skills
- Improves body composition in all age groups, helps delay the aging process

Psychological

- Releases stress and increases job productivity
- Increases our self-esteem, and the endorphins produced make us happy!

Cardiovascular Guidelines

According to the American College of Sports Medicine (ACSM), you should train 30 or 60 minutes three to five times a week. Between exercise sessions, you should rest from 36 to 48 hours to insure injury-free training and allow enough time for regeneration. For your cardiorespiratory system

least a 20 minute period. This activity could be biking, climb-

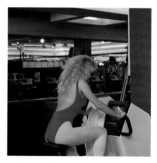

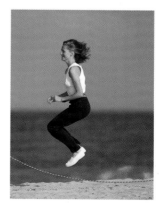

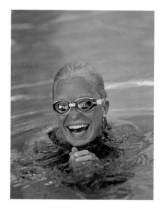

to reap benefits, you should perform a cardiovascular activity for at

ing stairs, rowing, jogging, walking, swimming, or cross-country skiing.

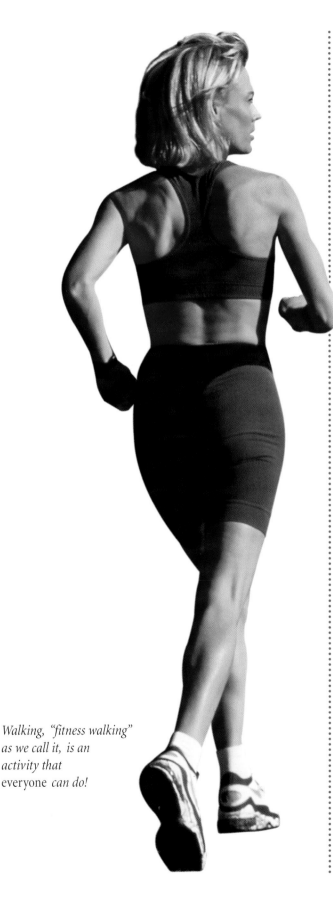

Walking, "fitness walking" as we call it, is an activity that everyone can do!

Walking

Walking is my absolute favorite activity. It is also the favorite among my personal training clients. The technique is easy to learn; you can do it outside or on a treadmill. In Germany, it took some convincing to show people the difference between "Wandern," which is a sort of hiking, and fitness walking. It took time, but we are slowly developing a nation of devoted walkers. In the USA, fitness enthusiasts walk in shopping centers for safety and weather reasons. The beauty of walking outdoors is the ability to breathe in oxygen in greater quantities. Of course, you must search out the quality, and that is usually away from the big cities.

Walking Technique

First, check your posture: shoulders depressed, chest held high, abdominals pulled together. Second, check foot technique. Keep toes straight in front, as if you were walking on a tight rope. Now strike with your heel first, roll up to the balls of your feet and then your toes. As the foot reaches the back of its stride, really *push off* with the ball of your foot. Your knees are relaxed and the length between your legs should be comfortable, i.e., just as you normally walk.

Third, let your arms swing naturally. Notice that the lead arm is opposite to the lead foot. Bring your forearms up so that your arms are in an L shape, keep this position and hold your arms close to your sides. Keep swinging your arms, but emphasize pulling the elbows backwards so you feel the muscles work in your upper back. Don't drop your forearms, and don't rotate your trunk—keep it straight and strong.

Exercise Prescription for Walking

Start walking everywhere. Try to use the above technique. If you are embarrassed to use the arms, then just swing them naturally and practice the foot technique. Now arrange a little time each day, 20–30 minutes, of continuous walking, and gradually increase your time to 60 minutes. Your tempo should be enough to put you in about 60–75% of your maximum heart rate (see page 16). It's a great help to invest in a heart-rate monitor, as this is the best way to control your progress. If you can train on a treadmill, start slowly until you have mastered your walking technique and feel comfortable on the machine. Start with 2.5 miles an hour and gradually increase. I have people now walking 4.5 to 5 miles an hour, and in the beginning, they were self-acclaimed snails! Just make sure you aren't getting out of breath, or you are working anaerobically.

Cross Training

A great motivational tool is cross training. This term refers to a combination of different forms of exercise or fitness training elements. I find cross training an amazingly successful method of motivating my clients. Whether I'm working with a newcomer to exercise or a toughie, each finds benefits that only one form of training cannot give them. One type of cross training is the mixture all the fitness elements: endurance, strength and flexibility. Cross training for cardiovascular endurance can mean exercise mixtures of biking, walking and swimming, for example. The concept of cross training was born in the early 1980s as the Triathlon became more popular. The training of the three disciplines—running, biking and swimming—offered not only diversity, but helped former runners learn new techniques to improve endurance and to strengthen neglected muscles. Because of this, many of the competitors were protected from possible injury due to the one-sidedness of running. As the concept of cross training took hold, it spread to other sports; for example, tennis players began playing basketball and runners began biking. The end result was that most athletes noticed a vast improvement in their main sport, which was also due to better coordination. When your body is confronted with different motor activities, it develops better coordination in general.

Training Prescription

Cross training isn't just meant for top athletes. You can fit cross training into your daily life. For example, you can bike to work one day, walk the next. If the distance is impossible, then bike on the weekends or mix it with a Saturday bike tour, Sunday swimming at your local community center and Monday taking a long walk around an interesting shopping center!

In a fitness studio setting, it might be a cardio circuit—something I love to include in most training programs: 10–15 minutes walking on the treadmill, 10 minutes on the stepper, 10 minutes on the rowing machine, 10 minutes on a stationary bike, 10 minutes on a skywalker or other type of elliptical machine, and 10 minutes on a recumbent bike,.if one is available. This way my client has done 60 minutes of continuous cardiovascular exercise, has used all sorts of different muscles to accomplish it, and has not gotten bored with the workout because there is constant variety.

Circuit training is a wonderful fitness workout which can easily offer the possibility of cross training. In our club, I have a group fitness class, "Hard Body Circuit," which has a cardiovascular step-aerobics segment. In a circle there are 10 stations with an exercise for each muscle group! After 90 minutes of training, our members can round off their session with 30 minutes of stretching. A truly perfect 120 minutes of cross training—for endurance, muscle and flexibility!

Types of Workouts

I want to introduce you to some of the newer trends in fitness. Many have established themselves in our everyday fitness vocabulary; others might be new to you. A big tip from me for all the following workouts: It isn't how fast or how much you do that counts, it is how you do the workout. This means the right technique is that which really makes the difference. Fast most often means sloppy, sloppy means incorrect, incorrect means injury. Injuries don't happen right away; they are programmed by constant incorrect repetition.

Step Aerobics

Stepping up and down on an adjustable platform was popularized by the sport article company Reebok. At the end of the 1980's, they not only developed and marketed this type of workout, but also researched it before bringing to the general public. This was a first for any sport article company. I was present in Toronto, when they proclaimed their new step training to be as important as running, tennis and basketball. A proud moment in the life of a fitness

Different Types of Cardiovascular Training

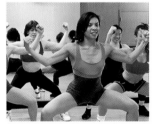

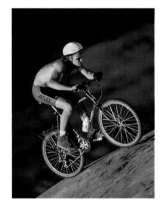

The heart is our most important muscle.

combination of aerobics exercise and biking or running.

If the classic high-low or low-impact class is not your thing, then try spinning or step aerobics.

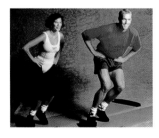

The preventative aspect of cardiovascular training is of greatest importance. The best form of general cardio-vascular training is a

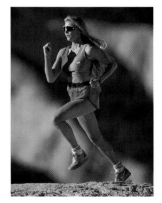

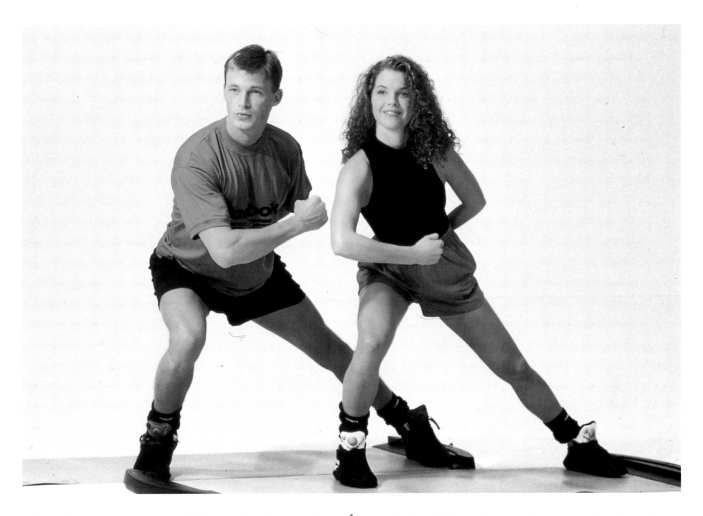

A form of training that really works the legs without impact. Great for preparing for the winter sports season.

Slide aerobics is a really athletic workout form. You glide across a special mat while wearing special socks that slip over your shoes. Bumpers or ramps at each end of the mat insure proper foot placement. It's important, in slide training, not to overdo—a little goes a long way. For cross training and preparatory training for winter sports, it is very valuable. It's also a great tool for muscle training, especially in the area of post rehabilitation.

professional! This workout was based on training in track and field, where athletes had to run up steps. It was refined, set to the correct speed of music, and each step pattern was given a special name. Guidelines were set down for safe and effective training. This workout is not only efficient cardiovascular training, but works arms and legs muscularly as well. Reebok developed eight subsequent programs in step training to meet the progressive needs of its participants.

In the basic program, or "step intro" as it is called, you learn the basic steps and their names. Of greatest importance is step technique. The foot is placed heel first in the middle of the platform (this way you get a better workout in the gluteals and you don't stamp your foot on the platform, avoiding unneeded impact). You roll your foot up onto the platform, and when you step down, you roll down toe, ball, heel, without *bouncing* (a very common mistake). As with all group fitness aerobic workouts, you should learn to use your feet properly before bringing your arms into it.

My recommended music tempo is 118 to 126 bpm (beats per minute)—unfortunately, most instructors teach far faster!

Adjust step height to your height (one or two are usually fine, three steps if you're a basketball player!).

Slide Aerobics

Sliding looks easy enough, but it's important to learn the correct technique right from the beginning and to stay in the basic moves for a longer period of time. Men especially love this simple and athletic workout. Developed from dry training for speed skaters, this workout form really exercises the adductors and abductors, i.e., inside and outside of the thigh. Simple arm movements are included which strengthen and challenge the upper-body muscles.

Indoor Stationary Cycling (Spinning)

This extremely popular, relatively new form of group fitness training is easily done alone. I have all my personal training clients "Spinning"! What *is* this phenomenon? Stationary biking to music! This incredible workout was developed by a man called Johnny G., a South African biking freak who crossed the USA in record time through strength, will, and imagery. He took his experience and turned it into a fantastic workout that almost any healthy person can do. It is imperative to wear a heart-rate monitor while doing this class. In this way the teacher and you can control your intensity level. Just as in step, many subsequent forms of indoor or stationary biking have been developed. In its true form, it should remain an athletic workout, imitating real biking techniques. In time, this cardiovascular exercise will really help lower your resting heart rate Just make sure you get a good teacher and wear and use your heart-rate monitor!

Watch Your Intensity

Nothing is worse for a beginner than to start off with too much intensity. It's a surefire way to quickly become discouraged, and disenchanted with continuing a fitness program. So, you people out there who train often but don't seem to be getting anywhere, heed my advice.

Also, a big tip—take enough time to warm up. Start each cardiovascular exercise with an adequate warm-up (at least 6 minutes of low-intensity work). If you're jogging or running on a treadmill, walk at a brisk pace for 6 minutes, *then* run—you'll be able to run longer! Now for some specifics:

● **Breathing**

If your breathing becomes rapid and you can only breathe in and out of your mouth (panting), then slow your pace down.

● **Perspiration**

It's normal and healthy to sweat! When you first start working out, you might either sweat enormously or hardly at all; with time it should normalize. If you sweat abnormally, or work out heavily and don't sweat at all, it's time to visit the doctor! Just remember to hydrate (drink enough during your workouts and afterward).

● **Technique**

If you start stumbling over your step or tripping when walking, it's a warning sign that you're tired and are unable to focus or con-

centrate. Remember, technique is the key to success. You need to concentrate on your movements for your movements to bring your body to where it should be.

● **Motivation**

If your motivation wanes during a class or session, it could be because you are tired or distracted, or simply that the teacher is not instructing the class correctly. The choreography might be too complicated because the teacher does not build it up logically, in easy-to-follow sequences. Many instructors don't really know how to work with the music. It can be a real motivation killer, if you feel the rhythm and beats and the instructor isn't working within the phrasing of the music, or the music is blah! But, if you are working out alone, you are your own DJ. Drop your favorite CD or cassette in your player and go for it! There is nothing like inspiring music to give us the power to work out just a little bit longer. If you're on a treadmill and have set your goal for 20 minutes, but wane after 10, tell yourself "just one more song, then I'll stop." Go for the next song and then the next. Magic, you have 20 minutes!

Home Equipment

As more and more people turn to personal trainers, many exercisers want to invest in their own equipment. It's not easy to know what to buy or what brand to choose. If you have a personal trainer, let him or her help you with your selection. Here are a few hints on which investments are best:

● If you have room and can invest the money, a good treadmill is a good start. You can walk or jog, so it serves two functions. There are some excellent home treadmills on the market. Many of them even fold up, so they are space saving. Just make sure they are stable and have good cushioning.

● An ergometer or stationary bike is also a great investment. You could even buy a "spinning" bike if you want something that simulates a real bike.

● A rowing machine is also a good investment, but it is important to use the proper technique to spare you back misery.

● Ab-shapers, for performing correct abdominal exercises, are not too expensive and often a good reminder to exercise that body part daily!

● If space is not a problem in your home, you might want to invest in a so-called "station;" a mini-fitness center. You would have lat pull, butterfly, chest press, leg extension and flexion, biceps and triceps training, all in one set-up. Before you invest in something like this, it's important to know which ones available are technologically good. For this, you need expert advice.

● Free weights should *definitely* be included in your selection.

Before you go out and equip yourself with everything you think you need, work-out with less first. Make sure the equipment will actually be used, before investing in it.

Finding the Right Fitness Center

● Always visit the fitness center, don't go by what someone tells you or by just telephoning. The atmosphere of the club must feel right to you. Look at the clientele: are they the types of people you want to sit in a sauna with?

● If you have no experience with fitness centers, consult some friends who have had experience. Let them give you some tips.

● What kind of equipment does the club have? There should be a good selection of cardiovascular equipment, like treadmills, ergometers (bikes), rowing machines, steppers, and recumbent bikes. The new elliptical machines are great!. They should have a good selection of strength-training machines, one for each body part, and free weights. They should have an area in the fitness section for stretching and perhaps one for abdominal training.

● Do they have a sauna and/or steam bath? Really examine the spa area. Is it hygienic?

● Is the studio staff friendly and helpful? Did they show you the whole studio and explain everything clearly?

● What kind of education do the trainers have? Do they have a degree in sports education? Do the aerobic or group fitness instructors have training beyond just theoretical certification?

● Do the trainers attend continuing education courses and work-shops regularly?

● What kinds of group fitness classes are offered? Are the class descriptions clear and do the descriptions really fit what is going on inside the room? Do the group-fitness (aerobics) rooms have special flooring? (Best are wood with special under-floor construc-tion to absorb impact.) Is there adequate ventilation, including air-conditioning?

● Do they offer personal training? What kind of qualifications do their personal trainers have? (An ex-dancer is not necessarily a qualified personal trainer, for example!) They need to have been educated in personal training technique.

● Is the whole club well looked-after? Are the floors clean? Is the equipment cared for? Make sure it isn't rusty or layered with old sweat!

● Are there enough lockers? You'll want to stow your valuables. How are the showers? Look at the sauna and steam room. Will you feel good sitting in there?

● Ask for a trial class or trial workout in the fitness area. Was the trainer helpful? Did he or she correct you? Were his or her di-rections and instructions clear and to the point? Did he or she answer your questions adequately?

Once you get back home, add up all the good and bad points and then decide what the most important criteria are for you. If you are not sure, visit the club a second time. There may be things you missed. Don't let anyone pressure you into joining, the club won't be gone tomorrow. Turn it over in your head and compare what you have seen with other offers.

When visiting a center make sure that the staff is knowledgeable and will be able to advise you correctly.

the instructor should correct participants, and give instructions clearly and precisely. Consult the group fitness

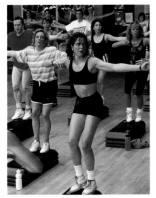

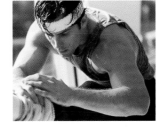

instructor or trainer with any difficulties. A competent trainer will welcome your questions.

Never begin a training program in a club by yourself. The staff should clearly show you the techniques and correct your execution of the movements—not show you a machine and go on to the next one without your having the chance to try them. In fitness classes, also,

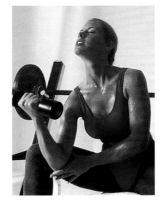

VI. The Training Plans

Here are several plans for different lifestyles, but before each training session, it is absolutely important to warm up! Warming up prepares your body both physiologically and psychologically for the oncoming intensity. A properly constructed and timed warm-up is especially important for the prevention of injury to our skeletal and muscle systems.

An active warm-up is the best way to activate the circulation of blood in our body, as well as raise our body temperature. Sitting in a sauna or rubbing yourself down with massage oil are *not* what warming up is all about. (Yes, I've seen women with sweatsuits and sport shoes in the sauna "warming up"! Men, it seems, are no smarter, having been discovered warming up in *their* saunas!) Warming up also *actively* helps the cardiovascular system prepare itself for the oncoming workout by slowly raising our heart rate and allowing our lungs to economize on the consumption of oxygen. On top of all this, our coordinative ability also becomes fine-tuned and our psyche has a chance to get used to the idea of exercising!

A Proper Warm-Up

If you are starting an exercise program for the very first time, or you're out of condition, it's best to begin with easy walking, or walking in place if you're inside. Try to spend 6 or 7 minutes doing this. Round it out with appropriate stretches (also called pre-stretches).

If you have more time, or feel you would like to extend your warm-up, by all means do so. Usually, I have my clients warm up for 10 to 15 minutes, depending on their schedule. All forms of non-impact endurance activity are recommended, such as biking, walking or stepping—these activities also on stationary equipment—or swimming, or just moving gently to music.

Begin the warm-up with low intensity and gradually but continually increase your level. You should feel your joints loosening and a warmth flowing through your body. It takes about 6 minutes for the synovial fluid (fluid that lubricates the joints) to go from a somewhat gelatinous state to a fluid state.

To prepare psychologically and because it feels good after a tense day, you may round off the cardiovascular section of the warm-up with stretches, for those body parts to be exercised. Check in the exercise section for the stretch exercises corresponding to the muscle group to be used, but pre-stretches,

An active warm-up gets your circulation moving and prepares you for the oncoming workout. My exercises take very little time and are designed so they can be carried out anywhere—use small bottles from the hotel minibar instead of hand weights. At home, grab a broom handle. Take a bicycle pump to your office.

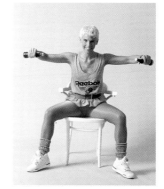

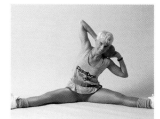

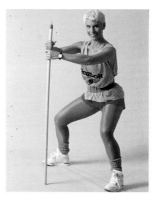

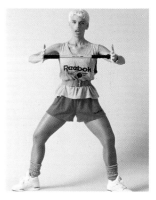

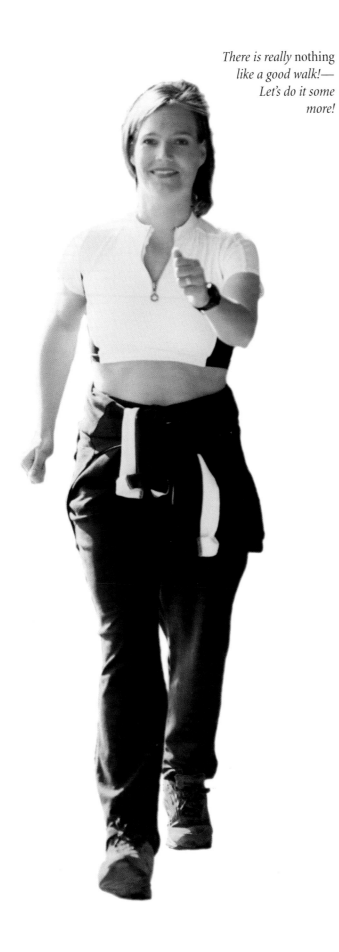

There is really nothing like a good walk!— Let's do it some more!

as they're called in fitness circles, are held for a shorter time, 8 to 10 seconds. These stretches are not aimed at increasing flexibility. They are just considered a psychological preparation for the work to come. I tell my clients to "free" their muscles.

After warming up, exercising will be a lot easier. You'll begin your training session with élan and energy.

Using the Training Plans

In the following section, you'll find seven different training plans that have already been introduced to you in chapter II. If my description at the beginning of each plan fits you and your lifestyle —you can start right away! If you find, however, that you and your lifestyle encompass a combination of factors, combine several plans and utilize exercises specially geared to overcoming your weaknesses. Remember, these training recommendations have been conceived and developed as a basic plan. As you progress, you can individualize your own training workouts by combining exercises, adding more repetitions or more sets, using stronger tubing, heavier weights, etc.

Important Information

In each training plan you'll receive the following "exercise prescription":

- **training goal—what you're aiming for**
- **where you can train**
- **type of equipment**
- **exercise schedule**
- **cardiovascular endurance training tips**
- **warm-up tips**
- **muscle and stretching exercises for upper body/lower body/trunk**

Exercise instructions are given in chapter IV, divided under the various body parts. Training plans refer, for example, to Chest: Ex. 1, 3. You then simply look in the Chest section of chapter IV for exercises 1 and 3 to find instructions, explanations, and appropriate photos.

- **exercise tips, additional information, encouragement, helpful reminders.**

Training Plan: Office Prisoners

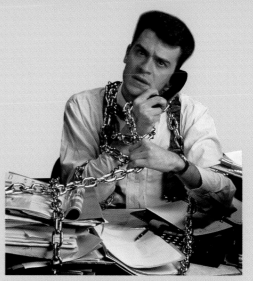

Are you an office prisoner? Do you sit for hours working at your computer and/or desk? Sitting 6 to 8 hours a day in place will not only tighten but weaken your back muscles.

Training Goal	Strengthen back and chest muscles, improve posture and circulation
Place	Office
Equipment	Rubber bands, tubing, books, bottles, chair, wall
Frequency	At least once a day; better, exercises for upper body, particularly stretching exercises, up to 3× a day, especially if you sit more than 6 hours a day. The whole training program 2–3× a week.

Cardiovascular Training

Use stairs instead of elevator or escalator. If you can manage it, take a 10-minute walk during your lunch hour. A little fresh air alone can rejuvenate—concentrate on your breathing technique.

Warm-Up

If you don't have time for a full warm-up (see page 126), at least do the following:
Sitting or standing: 8–10× shoulder-rolls, 8× lift and lower your shoulders.
Standing: Walk or march in place 5 minutes, add some door squats (p. 94, ex. 5).
Shake out your arms and legs.

Upper Body

Training

Shoulders	Ex. 5 (shoulder, biceps, abs)
Chest	Ex. 1 (standing, sitting), 3 (with a partner), 10
Triceps	Ex. 4 (use a book or bottle instead of tubing)
Upper Back	Ex. 1 (use a bodybar or pole), 2, 3 (Advanced: with stronger tubing or an expander), 7, 10 (use books or small bottles as weights)

Stretches

Shoulders	Ex. 10
Chest	Ex. 11, 12, 13 (repeat exercise more often)
Triceps	Ex. 6
Upper Back	Ex. 13, 16

Lower Body

Training

Buttocks	Ex. 5 (also for quadriceps)
Quadriceps	Ex. 1 (Advanced: with rubber bands)
Hamstrings	Ex. 12 (Advanced: with rubber bands)
Calves	Ex. 7

Stretches

Buttocks	Ex. 7 (sitting)
Quadriceps	Ex. 9
Hamstrings	Ex. 17 (If you are not flexible, begin with leg on a low platform or object, increase height with flexibility)
Calves	Ex. 9

Tip

Constant sitting tightens and weakens our back muscles. Remedy this by always sitting up straight. Pull your shoulder blades down and together. In this way, you will automatically strengthen your back muscles.

Trunk

Training

Abs	Ex. 13 (also for shoulder muscles)
Lower Back	Ex. 1 (Instead of lying down, "rock" while standing with your back to a wall)

Stretches

Lower Back	Ex. 8 (Instead of sitting on the floor, sit on the edge of a chair. Hold your hands behind your knees, or instead of a partner hold onto the door frame.)

Training Plan: Standing for Hours

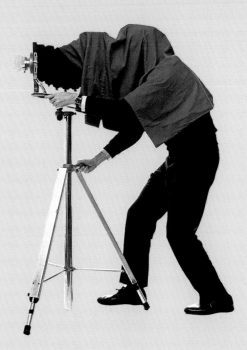

Do you work in a profession where you have to be standing still, on your feet, all day long? Then this is the right plan for you.

Training Goal	Stabilize trunk, strengthen back, improve posture, mobilize foot and calf muscles
Place	At home (in the morning before work or in the evening); but many exercises can be done while at work or during breaks
Equipment	Small weights, tubing, rubber bands, own body weight
Frequency	2–3× a week, abs trained daily

Exercises you can do as you are standing, while on the job, not only help to strengthen muscles but also relax them. Stretching these parts of the body is essential in reaching your goal.

Cardiovascular Training

I suggest cycling. Bike instead of drive. Because you stand all day, it's nice to sit *and* get a great workout.

Warm-Up

Try to start with walking or cycling (about 15 minutes). If this is impossible for you, here are some other alternatives:
- **Stand up and sit down in a chair 20–30×, 3 sets.**
- **Do door squats (p. 94, ex. 5).**
- **Sitting or standing: 8–10× shoulder-rolls, 8× lift and lower your shoulders.**
- **Sitting: Lift and lower your heels (calf raises) 20× both feet, 10× alternating feet.**
- **Lift toes, keep heels on the floor, 20× both feet, 10× alternating feet.**

Upper Body

Training
Shoulders   Ex. 1, 2
Upper Back   Ex. 2, 3, 11, 12

Stretching
Shoulders   Ex. 10
Upper Back   Ex. 13, 16, 17

Lower Body

Training
Buttocks   Ex. 5
Quadriceps   Ex. 2, 7, 8 (to mobilize, also trains abductors)
Hamstrings   Ex. 12
Calves   Ex. 3, 4, 8 (Do exercise on the stairs; holding onto the banisters)

Stretching
Buttocks   Ex. 6, 8
Quadriceps   Ex. 9, 11
Hamstrings   Ex. 16, 17
Adductors   Ex. 21
Abductors   Ex. 22
Calves   Ex. 9 and stretching ex. 8 (use stairs, hold onto the banisters)

Tip

Divide up your training into body parts. Upper body for the morning break. Lower body later in the day.
If you have stairs at work, do some calf stretches on one of your trips up or down the stairs.
Be constantly aware of your posture
Consciously press your shoulders down.
It is important that you put your legs up as often as possible.

Trunk

Training
Abs   Ex. 3, 4 ,7, 8, 9, 13 (also for shoulder muscles)
Lower Back   Ex. 1 (also standing with back to the wall), 2, 4

Stretching
Lower Back   Ex. 6, 7, 8 (If without a partner, hold onto an immovable object.)

Training Plan:
On the Go? No Excuses!

Are you often on the road—traveling, on business trips, in hotels—and find yourself saying you have no time and no place to exercise? Now, this "No Excuses!" workout plan is just for you!

Training Goal	Training for the whole body, muscular strength and cardiovascular conditioning
Place	Hotel room, train, airplane, automobile
Equipment	Rubber bands, tubing, suitcase, little bottles
Frequency	At least 2× weekly (1 exercise for each body part each training day); 3× weekly, 1–2 exercises for each body part)

If you want to train more than 3 times a week, leave 24 hours between exercises of certain muscles. Always try to train "partner muscles" in one workout session, e.g. back/abs, biceps/triceps, quadriceps/biceps femoris. And the good news is: You can train your abs daily!

Cardiovascular Training

Use stairs instead of the elevator or walk up escalators. Even if your hotel room is on the 30th floor, you can leave the elevator on the 26th floor, for example, and walk up the rest of the way—"No excuses!"

Warm-Up

Choose a warm-up that really gets your circulation going. In a hotel, use its pool or gym. Walk on a treadmill, or up 10 flights of stairs *slowly*! If that's not possible, try this:
   Sitting or standing : 8-10× shoulder rolls, 8× lift and lower your shoulders.
   Stand up and sit down in a chair 20–30×. Alternate this with door squats (p. 94, ex. 5).
   Before leg exercises: 8–20× alternate lifting and lowering your heels.

Upper Body

Training

Shoulders	Ex. 5 (Advanced), 7 (also with a suitcase)
Chest	9 (Advanced), 10 (Beginners)
Biceps	Ex. 1, 2, 4, (with bottles instead of weights), 6
Triceps	Ex. 1, 2, 3
Upper Back	Ex. 2, 3, 7, 10 (with smaller bottles as weights), 12 (with suitcase)

Stretching

Shoulders	Ex. 10
Chest	Ex. 11, 12, 13,
Biceps/Triceps	Ex. 6 (triceps)
Upper Back	Ex. 13, 16

Lower Body

Training

Buttocks	Ex. 5 (on doors and car doors)
Quadriceps	Ex. 1, 2 (also with a chair), 3
Hamstrings	Ex. 12 (Advanced: with rubber bands or ankle weights)
Calves	Ex. 6, 7 (you can also use books as weights)

Stretching

Buttocks	Ex. 7 (sitting)
Quadriceps	Ex. 9
Hamstrings	Ex. 14 or 17
Calves	Ex. 9

Tip

Train in your hotel room, either in the morning after taking a shower or in the evening before you go out or to bed. You can train your upper body while sitting on an airplane or on a train, even as a passenger in a car—so there's really "no excuses" anymore not to get in shape.

Trunk

Training

Abs	Ex. 1, 5, 7, 12 (Advanced), 13
Lower Back	Ex. 2, 3, 5

Stretching

Lower Back	Ex. 6, 8

Training Plan: Toughies

Are you a sports freak? Do you play tennis, run marathons, and love mountain biking? Or maybe you teach 15 aerobic classes a week? This plan is for people who need to find balance in their lives. Regenerative training is important for you.

Training Goal	To restore balance to overused muscles, and strengthen weaker ones that have suffered from one-sided training; cross training, flexibility
Place	At home, fitness center, outside
Equipment	Small weights, tubing, ball, rope, punching bag, free weights.
Frequency	At least 1× a week; in every unit you should train with the same intensity to keep up the same level.

Cardiovascular Training

3–15 minutes of jumping rope, 3–5 minutes of front lunges (quadriceps ex. 7 or 8); 3–5 minutes boxing on the punching bag
Low-intensity, long-duration walking, at 60–70% of maximum heart rate

Warm-Up

Choose walking or cycling. Start with slow intensity, increase steadily.
Mobilize joints: shoulder, hip and knee, and stretch if you want to (hold stretches 10 seconds or a little longer if you need to). If you plan to do your cardiovascular workout after the warm-up, leave off stretches, otherwise your heart rate will fall too low.

Upper Body

Training

Shoulders	Ex. 2, 3, 9
Chest	Ex. 5, 6, 9
Biceps	Ex. 1, 2, 4, 5*
Triceps	Ex. 1, 2, 3
Upper Back	Ex. 2, 3*, 8, 9

Stretching

Shoulders	Ex. 10
Chest	Ex. 11, 12
Biceps/Triceps	Ex. 6 (triceps)
Upper Back	Ex. 13, 16, 17

Info

When you train sport-specific, you are aiming for speed and agility. This program is designed to bring your body back into balance, therefore all movements should be slow and controlled.

Lower Body

Training

Buttocks	Ex. 2, 4
Quadriceps	Ex. 1, 2, 3, 7
Hamstrings	Ex. 13, 14 (definitely with a bodybar)
Abductors	Ex. 18, 19
Abductors	Ex. 18
Calves	Ex. 3, 4

Stretching

Buttocks	Ex. 7
Quadriceps	Ex. 9, 10, 11
Hamstrings	Ex. 16, 17
Adductors/	
Abductors	Ex. 23
Calves	Ex. 7 (as a variation of stretching)

Tip

If you have the feeling that one arm, or body part, is weaker than the other, concentrate on building up that particular arm at the beginning of your training. Exercises for that purpose are specially marked here, with a *. When both arms or body parts are of equal strength, you can then begin to exercise both at the same level.

Trunk

Training

Abs	Ex. 2, 5, 6, 11, 12
Lower Back	Ex. 4, 5

Stretching

Lower Back	Ex. 7, 8

Training Plan:
Models and
New Moms

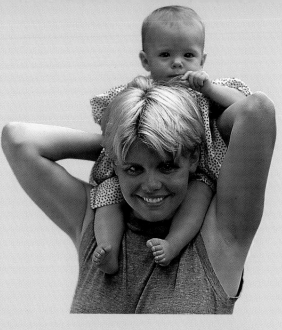

You just had a baby and want to get fit again? You're slim, but still feel "flabby"? You've decided to do something about that unsightly cellulite? Here's a workout for you.

Training Goal	Firm the body in general without building up too much muscle mass; emphasis on triceps, abs, buttocks, adductors, abductors, quadriceps, hamstrings. Reduction of body fat.
Place	At home
Equipment	Tubing, small weights, rubber bands
Frequency	Frequency: 2–3× a week for fat burning, at least 3× a week cardiovascular.

TLC: Young mothers should start training with a low intensity. Be conscious of consequences and do not overdo. To promote circulation in the legs, buttocks and arms, rub them with a good massage oil after showering or bathing. Always use body lotion or oil after showering in order to keep skin supple and well hydrated.

Cardiovascular Training

Start your cardio training with low intensity (55–65% of maximum heart rate), e.g., walking in place 5–10 minutes. Increase training slowly to 30–40 minutes.

Warm-Up

Sitting or standing: 8–10× shoulder-rolls, 8× lift and lower your shoulders.
Standing: While walking 5 minutes in place, shake your arms and legs out.
Sitting: Lift and lower your heels, alternating feet.

Upper Body

Training

Shoulders	Ex. 1, 7, 8
Chest	Ex. 2, 4, 9A, 10 (at the beginning)
Biceps	Ex. 3, 5, 6
Triceps	Ex. 2, 3, 4, 5
Upper Back	Ex. 9 (without weights)

Stretching

Shoulders	Ex. 10
Chest	Ex. 11, 12, 13
Biceps/Triceps	Ex. 6 (triceps)
Upper Back	Ex. 13, 15

Info

Women tend to neglect training their upper body. It is not only muscularly important, it balances out the lower body, both structurally and harmoniously.

Lower Body

Training

Buttocks	Ex. 1, 2, 3, 5
Quadriceps	Ex. 2, 3
Hamstrings	Ex. 14
Adductors/ Abductors	Ex. 18, 20
Calves	Ex. 1, 2

Stretching

Buttocks	Ex. 6, 8
Quadriceps	Ex. 10
Adductors/ Abductors	Ex. 21, 24
Hamstrings	Ex. 16, 17
Calves	Ex. 9

Tip

It is better to train for a longer period in a lower intensity (walking 30 minutes and longer, for example) than vice versa. This is a much more effective way to burn fat when you are not in condition (p.20). If you want to take part in group fitness classes, choose a so-called "fatburner" program. It is important, however, for you to avoid all high-impact movements.

Trunk

Training

Abs	Ex. 1, 3, 7, 8, 9,11
Lower Back	Ex. 1, 3, 5

Stretching

Lower Back	Ex. 6, 7

Training Plan: Hip Hop Kids

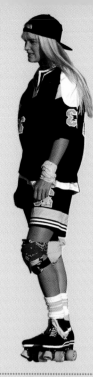

This is goal-oriented training for young people with concentration and postural problems.

Training Goal	Body-awareness training with low-intensity strength and cardio exercises; cardiovascular conditioning and coordination will be increased through fun-to-do interval training.
Place	At home, in a club, with friends, in school
Equipment	Bodybar, own body weight
Frequency	2–3× a week

Circulatory and Endurance Training

Walk/Run: Work out up to one hour. Alternate between 10 minutes walking, 2 minutes running, repeat 4×. Build up to 20-minute walk, 10-minute run, repeat 2×. On other days, burn-fat walk or cycle 30–60 minutes. If you have less time available, try 3–15 minutes jumping rope and 10 minutes walking.

Cardiovascular Training

Try to walk at a tempo of 3, 4, or 5 miles per hour; or cycling—change between 15 minutes fast and 15 minutes slow—or in-line skating.

Warm-Up

Choose two of your favorite songs, and move to the music freestyle (as if you were in a disco). Let the music get inside you and tell you what moves to do!

Upper Body

Training

Shoulders	Ex. 5, 8 (your partner trains lats, you train shoulders)
Chest	Ex. 3, 10
Biceps	Ex. 6
Triceps	Ex. 1
Upper Back	Ex. 5

Stretching

Shoulders	Ex. 10
Chest	Ex. 14
Biceps/Triceps	Ex. 6 (triceps)
Upper Back	Ex. 14

Lower Body

Training

Quadriceps	Ex. 4, 5, 6, 8
Hamstrings	Ex. 5, 15

Stretching

Quadriceps	Ex. 9
Hamstrings	Ex. 16

Important: Try to be outside in the fresh air as much as possible.

Cycling, jogging, and in-line skating train your leg muscles.

Tip

If you have a friend who is also interested in getting fit, work out together. And don't forget to tune in to your favorite radio station, or put on your favorite CD or tape. Music makes everything easier, especially if you're going it alone.

Trunk

Training

Abs	Ex. 4 (without tubing)
Lower Back	Ex. 3

Stretching

Lower Back	Ex. 8 (with a partner if possible)

Training Plan: Couch Potatoes

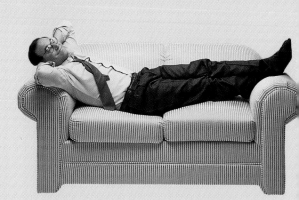

After sitting in an office all day, do you tend to just lie around when you come home? This program is aimed at you inactive, uninspired millions whose training goal is really just to get off the couch and away from the television set!

Training Goal	Complete body training, especially for the cardiovascular system. More energy, flexibility and muscular endurance is the objective.
Place	At home or outside...also in front of the TV!
Equipment:	Tubing, own body weight
Frequency	At least 2× a week

Begin by realizing that even a little is better than nothing at all! Most exercises can also be done in front of the TV. Your abs can be trained daily.

Cardiovascular Training

Start with a 10-minute walk outside in the fresh air; increase time gradually. Walk up stairs every time you get a chance. Train muscle strength 2–3× a week, 10 minutes or longer.

Warm-Up

Walk in place 5–10 minutes, swing your arms naturally.
Sitting or standing: 8–10× shoulder rolls, first backwards, repeat forwards; 8× lift and lower your shoulders.
Sitting: Lifting and lowering your heels, alternate feet.

Upper Body

Training

Shoulders	Ex. 7 (also with a book)
Chest	Ex. 10 (at the beginning), 9 (later)
Biceps	Ex. 4
Triceps	Ex. 1
Upper Back	Ex. 1, 10

Stretching

Shoulders	Ex. 10
Chest	Ex. 13
Biceps/Triceps	Ex. 6 (triceps)
Upper Back	Ex. 17

Lower Body

Training

Buttocks	Ex. 3, 5
Quadriceps	Ex. 1
Hamstrings	Ex. 14
Adductors/ Abductors	Ex. 20
Calves	Ex. 7

Stretching

Buttocks	Ex. 7, 8
Quadriceps	Ex. 10
Hamstrings	Ex. 16
Adductors/ Abductors	Ex. 22
Calves	Ex. 9

Tip

If you haven't moved
your body in years,
it's *very*
hard to start.
But try to force yourself
up and outside to get
some fresh air at least
10 minutes a day.
Instead of waiting around for
and taking the elevator,
use the stairs.
At the beginning,
it's enough just to walk
a few flights; you'll soon
get the hang of it.

Trunk

Training

Abs	Ex. 1, 7, 9
Lower Back	Ex. 1, 3, 6

Stretching

Lower Back	Ex. 6, 7

VII. Nutrition

"Once upon a time, when I was a pear..."
I had ended my 400,000th diet. That was back in
1985. I had rigorously followed the Beverly Hills
Diet and had lost more than 20 pounds in six weeks.
To my horror and dismay (why should I have been
surprised? it had happened "oh so many times"
before), I gained back 25 pounds in an even shorter
space of time. That was *it*!

My entire life had been a succession of diets. At least it seemed that way. When I was 10 years old, I began with liquid diets. My school locker was filled with cans of the stuff! Sugar was considered poison in our house. Mom used artificial sweetener for everything. We ate diet cookies, diet chocolate; I even had a diet birthday cake once. Mom was always on a diet so—like mother like daughter—so was I.

"Real" food was foreign to me until I came to Europe. When I let my guard down, I could almost enjoy food. I ate potatoes, hearty breads and incredible cakes and pastries. In between "real" food, I continued the starve-and-stuff syndrome, until 1985.

A Vicious Circle
After the disappointment of the Beverly Hills Diet, I saw with incredible clarity the cycle of losing and gaining weight…a vicious circle. I knew that, if I didn't change the way I thought and the way I was living, I would be paralyzed by this forever. I realized that I had never really lived life. I constantly based my goals on the state of my body, living for a future that would never come. "I'll wear this when I get thin, I'll do this or that when I'm thin, I will be more liked, more loved when I'm thin."

It was then, that I made a conscious decision to accept myself as I was and enjoy life and food, even if it meant being fat.

Eat Well and Feel Good
Stress at work, the strain of sports—for your body to be resilient it needs an optimal supply of nutrients. This only works with a sensible diet of the widest possible variety. Forget the frustration of dieting and having a guilty conscience. Your new strategy is: Consciously enjoy!

No single food on earth contains all the nutrients our bodies need. It takes the proper combination of different foods to cover the daily adult nutritional requirements: carbohydrates, fats, protein (for producing and maintaining energy), vitamins and minerals (to regulate metabolism and maintain health).

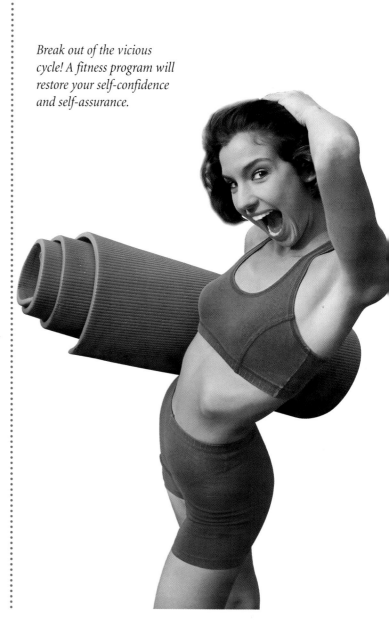

Break out of the vicious cycle! A fitness program will restore your self-confidence and self-assurance.

Carbohydrates: The High-Octane Fuel

Carbohydrates are the most important nutrient for active people and anyone who wants to eat right. Often maligned in the past as being fattening, now they are regarded as a health food. Carbohydrates are what provide the fast economical supply of energy that the muscles need.

And what about much-touted glucose that is supposed to immediately replace depleted energy? True, glucose is quickly absorbed into the blood and then is converted into energy right away. But beyond that, simple carbohydrates like sugar provide only calories, no vitamins or minerals. If you want to eat right, you should choose pasta, whole grain bread, potatoes, rice, cereal, legumes, vegetables and fruit. These foods contain complex carbohydrates. Since they are made up of several sugar molecules as opposed to sugar, they are absorbed slowly but steadily into the blood. This way, the blood sugar level remains constant and the body is fit longer. This spells the basis for endurance, concentration and coordination.

Proteins: The Body's Building Blocks

Protein is one of the main building blocks of all cells. It is indispensable to building and maintaining the body's overall mass as well as the muscles. Also, proteins are essential for producing enzymes (see nutritional terms, p. 152), hormones and antibodies.

The protein in meat is of especially high quality. Nowadays, most of us know it is healthier to forego red meat, if possible. High quality sources of vegetable protein are potatoes, legumes and grain products. In the right combination, vegetable proteins are easily comparable to meat. Some examples of ideal protein combinations are milk with grains (barley and buttermilk make a great soup) or legumes and grains (such as beans with corn). And, certainly, fish is an extremely healthy and flavorful source of protein. Tofu and soy products are also good choices.

Fats: The Calorie Bombs

Fat makes you fat. A single gram of fat provides nine calories, more than twice as much energy as a gram of carbohydrates. It is healthiest to consume one half of your fats, that is 35g, in the form of visible fat (such as oil, spreads, cooking fats) and the other half as hidden fats as contained in meat, sausage, cheese and baked goods. Aside from the amount, of course, the quality also plays a decisive role. The portion in your diet of saturated fats (in hydrogenated vegetable fats, meat and sausage), simple or monosaturated fats (in butter and olive oil) and polyunsaturated fats (in high-quality plant oils like safflower or corn oil) should each be one third.

Polyunsaturated fats are indispensable for your metabolism because the body can not produce them itself. They also lower

Your Daily Carbohydrate Allowance

About 55% to 60% of your energy intake should be in the form of carbohydrates. For 2,000 calories (the adult daily requirement) this would amount to close to 275 grams of carbohydrates. This is approximately the "food equivalent" of each of the following:

4 slices of bread
1 roll
1 banana
8 oz. potato
1½ oz. cereal
1 apple
1 teaspoon of honey
1 cinnamon roll
1 piece of candy

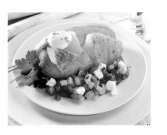
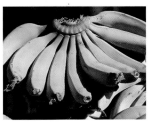
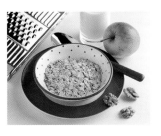

Carbohydrates and Fiber

Eating low-fat carbohydrates does something good for your body:

● Fiber, especially pectin and oat bran, help prevent heart attack.

●Fiber has a beneficial effect on the regulation of fat and cholesterol levels in the blood.

●Fiber protects the sensitive digestive tract.

your cholesterol level (see nutritional terms, p. 153). In addition, fat carries aroma, ensuring that food tastes good. And fat is what gives us the feeling of satiation after eating a meal.

Minerals: The Cramp Busters

A mineral deficiency, especially among active, athletic people, is no rarity. Little time for eating right or regular meals, stress at work, and day-to-day stress all magnify this lack. It comes out especially in stressful situations. Who hasn't had a sudden foot cramp that seems to come out of nowhere? The cause can be a mineral deficiency, especially a lack of potassium or magnesium.

However, setting sensible nutritional goals can help you prevent a mineral deficiency. For example, magnesium plays a key role in the interaction of nerves and muscles. A deficiency has been known to cause tremors and muscle cramps.

Magnesium and Calcium

It is impossible to get an oversupply of magnesium from natural sources. However, consult your doctor about magnesium supplements. This is important because overdoses of magnesium can interfere with absorption in the intestines of trace elements such as zinc. Increased susceptibility to infection results because zinc carries out vital functions in the immune system. An excess of magnesium can also account for the reduced absorption of calcium. Calcium, although in tiny amounts, is involved in muscle stimulation. Of course, its main job is building and maintaining teeth and bones. If there is a calcium deficiency, the body taps the calcium supply in the bones. This can cause bone brittleness and osteoporosis.

Did You Know

● Magnesium RDA (recommended daily allowance) for women is 280 milligrams per day; for men, 350 milligrams. Signs of magnesium deficiency are: muscle weakness, irritability and mental problems.

● Calcium RDA for adults, including women over age 50 on estrogen, are 1,000 milligrams per day. For women over 50 not on estrogen, all adults over 65, pregnant and lactating women and very sports-active people (my toughies), calcium intake should be 1,500 milligrams daily.

● Zinc RDA is 15 milligrams per day for men and 12 milligrams for women. Only 2 to 3 grams of zinc are present in the human body. All our cells contain zinc, but the highest concentrations are in bones, the prostate gland and the eyes! Too little zinc may result in delayed healing of wounds.

Proteins

Huge steaks for mega-muscles? Those times are long gone. Unless you're a professional athlete, you can manage fine without increased protein intake. The amounts of protein usually recommended range between slightly under to 0.5g per pound of body weight. For example, at a weight of 120 lbs. that would be about 50–60g per day, from taking in either:

4 oz. whole milk,
2 slices whole grain bread,
1 oz. Gouda cheese,
8 oz. potatoes,
1½ oz. nonfat yogurt
1¼ oz. oatmeal.

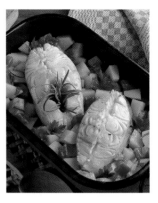

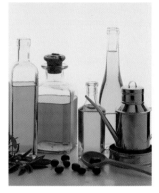

Fats

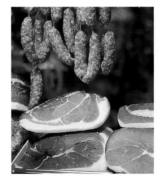

The body cannot survive without fat. For example, vitamins A, D and E can only be absorbed in combination with fat. Dietitians advise consuming 30% of your daily calorie allowance in the form of fat; one third should be unsaturated fat. That makes about 70g per day (1g fat = 9 cal.). People eat fat, mostly in the form of hidden fat, without realizing it. For example, there are 32g of fat in a hotdog, 30g in a chocolate bar and a whopping 42g in a large order of fries with mayonnaise. Cheese is the big culprit—so beware.

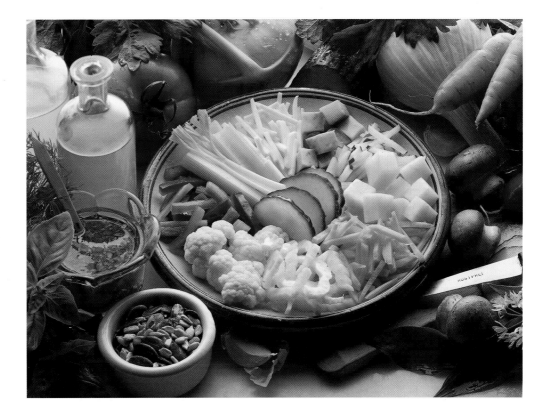

Vegetables are the best source of vitamins and minerals.

Minerals

Minerals play an important part not only in muscle contraction but also in building bones and regulating hydration. A lack of magnesium can cause muscle cramps.

Calcium deficiency has a negative influence on the health of bones and teeth.

Magnesium is plentiful in green vegetables such as broccoli, spinach and peas, as well as in whole grain products and legumes.

Dairy products of all types are a good source of calcium, but they are not always the best source if you have lactose intolerance. If this is the case turn to fish, broccoli, turnips and green leafy vegetables.

Electrolytes

Many sports drinks advertise the fact that they are fortified with electrolytes. When you drink them, you propably notice a slightly salty aftertaste. Electrolytes are actually salts that dissolve in water and can conduct electricity. They play an active role in body metabolism and functioning—they include potassium, sodium and the chlorides; to name a few. A deficiency or imbalance of electrolytes can occur as a result of illness, diarrhea, excessive perspiration (running a marathon and not drinking enough fluid containing electrolytes), vomiting, blood pressure medication or other drugs. It is of utmost importance that an electrolyte deficiency be treated quickly.

Sodium

Sodium, or common salt, is a leading food additive, both in factories and home cooking. After sugar, it is astounding how much salt is consumed in certain countries. I'm not just talking about the table salt that you sprinkle on your food. Almost all food products have long "shelf lives" due to extra added sodium. The products might have a long shelf life, but *you* won't if you don't watch your sodium consumption. Our bodies require less than 1,000 milligrams of sodium per day. The average American consumes between 3,000 to 6,000 miligrams of sodium per day! So watch it! By the way, when using table salt make it iodized salt, the richest dietary source of iodine.

Potassium

If you tend to perspire profusely, you especially need to watch both your sodium and your potassium intake. Both regulate the body's hydration and play an important role in contracting and relaxing the muscles. In general, we consume enough sodium, sometimes even too much, through salty food. A shortage of potassium is more likely to occur and can lead to muscle fatigue, circulatory problems or even cardiac muscle weakness. Good sources of potassium are fruit, especially bananas and apricots, potatoes and vegetables.

Iron

Especially among women, the supply of iron leaves something to be desired. This mineral is essential for transporting oxygen and for numerous enzyme systems. The need for iron increases with physical activity, since, on the one hand, oxygen consumption is very high, and on the other hand, a certain amount of iron is lost through perspiration. In addition, the iron loss in women through menstruation takes it toll. Iron deficiency leads to fatigue, lethargy and increased vulnerability to infections. Iron occurs mainly in meat, grains, legumes, vegetables, nuts and seeds. As a rule, the body can best utilize the iron contained in meat. Absorption of iron from plant foods can be enhanced by vitamin C. Eat a salad containing vitamin C or drink orange juice with meals. In contrast, black tea and coffee inhibit iron absorption and should not be drunk with meals. Iron supplements can help in cases of acute iron deficiency. Talk to your doctor.

Vitamins: Your Metabolism's Jumpstarter

Without vitamins, your metabolism would grind to a halt: neither carbohydrates nor proteins or fats could be broken down. There are 13 vitamins that the body must receive to survive. Especially vitamin E, the carotenes (beta-carotene), and vitamin C have received much press recently as so-called antioxidants (see nutritional terms, p. 152) and cell protectors. They are said to considerably boost the immune system and play a part in combating cancer and heart attack.

This is why scientists have recently been urging us to take more of these vitamins: 200mg to 300mg of vitamin C, 15mg to 30mg of beta carotene and 30 mg to 60 mg of vitamin E.

Can vitamins enhance athletic performance? Unfortunately, the notion of "the more, the better" doesn't apply. Taking too many vitamins has nothing to do with increasing performance; in fact, in some cases, it can seriously damage your health. In principle, it is safe to assume that an overdose can never come from food alone. However, taking supplements without supervision can easily lead to actual vitamin poisoning, especially with the fat-soluble vitamins A and D. But also extremely high doses of water-soluble vitamin B complexes can cause side effects.

Survey of Protective Vitamins

Vitamin C in		mg
200g	red bell pepper, raw	280
200g	broccoli	228
200g	brussel sprouts	228
125g	black currants	225
100g	kohlrabi	192
200g	papaya	164
125g	strawberries	80
50ml	orange juice	78
1	orange	63
1	kiwi	57
1	lemon	42
50g	sauerkraut	30

Carotinoids in		mg
100g	dandelion leaves	15.8
200g	carrots	14.0
200g	kale	8.2
200g	red bell pepper, raw	7.6
50g	fennel	5.3
50g	mango	4.2
200g	pumpkin	4.0
100g	lamb's lettuce	3.9
200g	broccoli	3.8
200g	apricots	3.6
200g	chicory	2.6
150g	honeydew melon	2.6
100g	iceberg lettuce	1.3

Vitamin E		mg
1T	wheat germ oil	25.8
10g	wheat germ	11.7
150g	fennel	9.0
1T	safflower oil	6.6
20g	hazelnuts	5.2
20g	almonds	5.0
1T	corn oil	3.6
200g	kale	3.4
50g	whole grain cereal	3.3
20g	oatmeal	3.0
1	slice whole grain bread with sunflower seeds	1.8
50g	dandelion leaves	1.3

Calculations based on energy/nutritional values table by B. and H. Heseker in "Nutritional Values in Foods," Umschauverlag, Frankfurt on Main, 1993.

Never Diet Again!

Eat consciously and enjoy. Sadly, many women, and men, have virtually trained their bodies to gain weight by continuous dieting. As soon as the body receives less nourishment it sets its flame low, as in times of famine, and adjusts itself accordingly. It uses fewer calories, even later on, when the diet is over. In earlier times of starvation, this mechanism was life saving. Today, it only serves to make us fatter. Pounds on, pounds off, pounds on... There is only one way to overcome this yo-yo effect: forget the quick-fix diets where you really only lose water and not fat. Put an end to the diet doldrums! The point is maintaining your weight long-term and changing your eating habits for the long haul. Learn to enjoy deliberately and remember something all too often forgotten amid the endless calorie counting and the diet frenzy: your psyche is being fed as well!

Thin—A Word of Warning

Many times dieting can trigger a latent eating disorder. If you think about food all the time, if your life is ruled by eating or not eating, if you constantly give excuses to family and friends for strange eating patterns, then you might be headed for trouble. Try to be honest with yourself. Seek out professional help or a support group dealing with eating disorders.

Do you think you can balance overeating with purging, either by vomiting or using laxatives? You should realize that, by doing so, you are violently abusing your digestive processes. Over time you will not only create imbalances in your body, but produce physical effects that can range from disfiguring to fatal. Please, get help!

If you feel power in *not* eating or in eating in an overly controlled way and are drastically "underfat" (less than 13% body fat), you are anorexic. I've been there. I've done that! My saving grace was that I *knew* that I had a problem! Look into the mirror, then go deep inside yourself and ask yourself if you are "dying" to be thin. First, admit to yourself that there is something you cannot do alone. But there is someone that can help you—just reach out and search for the right therapy.

Choice, Not Chance

It's not only important what we eat, but also how we eat. You have to change your eating behavior for the long haul. Common sense usually tells us just what is good for our health. It says: "Eat low-fat, nutritional foods like whole grains, fruit and vegetables, and get enough fiber!" But instead, feelings often overcome common sense and win out in the form of a piece of cheesecake or a box of chocolates. Most people are completely unaware of what and how much they eat and when. If you want to change your eating habits, you have to recognize your mistakes.

I always recommend that my clients write down everything

Fiber, the Secret Slenderizer

Although indigestible, fiber offers amazing benefits for health and figure. First, it requires extensive chewing, therefore forcing you to eat more slowly. Fiber is filling and makes you feel satiated longer. It prevents cravings,

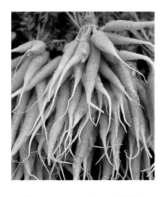

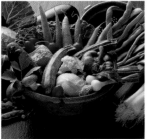

because fiber helps stabilize the level of blood sugar. Fiber activates intestinal function. Good digestion is the best basis for a good figure and healthy and glowing skin. Unfortunately, fiber is all too often neglected in most people's eating habits. Nutritionists recommend 30 grams per day. Half of this amount is already contained in

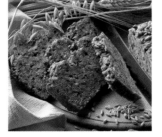

3 to 4 slices of whole grain bread. Plenty of raw veggies, legumes and fruit will balance the equation.

they eat for at least three days. Analyzing this record becomes part of the training plan. It is also important to consider: Did you eat because you were hungry, or because it tasted so good, or because you wanted to reward or distract yourself? Or did you just pig out on cookies all day and then go on to stuff yourself in a restaurant in the evening? Or did you munch a bunch of peanuts and chips in front of the TV? Become aware of your weaknesses and make a decision: Are you happy with the status quo or do you want to do something good for yourself? Are you willing to change some of your habits? Always remember that you are doing it for yourself. Not for your husband, your wife, your mother or your nutrition counselor/dietitian.

Once you have decided in favor of more conscious eating, then you need to realize that you can't change overnight. After all, it took years or decades to learn bad habits. Now, you have to eliminate your weaknesses step by step. Set yourself your personal goals and be patient with yourself.

Say Goodbye to Your Guilty Conscience

Many people have one thing in common: a sweet tooth. This preference is apparently something we are born with, as American studies of newborns have demonstrated. Blind tests on infants showed that all children love sweets. Sugar probably reminds them of the sweet flavor of mother's milk. So, accept your hankering for sweets, and learn to deal with it. If you're overcome by a craving for a candy bar, then eat just one—if you really want to! Don't devour it, but rather, enjoy it bite by bite. And remember: get rid of your guilty conscience! Instead, you should come to view it as completely normal to eat a candy bar now and then. That is much better than thinking all day about eating a candy bar and then "inhaling" a whole box of chocolate that evening.

The Balance of Energy: Your Calorie Account

The balance of energy is like a bank account: energy output and energy intake must remain in equilibrium just like receivables and expenditures, your positive and negative balance at the bank. Here, the currency is called calories (or joules) or kilocalories (or kilo-joules). Each gram of carbohydrates and protein equals about 4kcal (17kj), each gram of fat about 9 kcal (38kj,) and a gram of alcohol has 7kcal (30kj). Your energy needs are based on your basic metabolic rate (BMR) or the energy needed to maintain your bodily functions in a resting state) and the rate at which we expend energy during specific physical activities. Your stress rate varies according to your profession and leisure activities.

Of course, someone who is very active will need more. If you sit at a desk most of the time—as many of us do—as a woman you would need some 2,000 to 2,200 calories, as a man you would need somewhere between 2,400 and 2,600 calories. To maintain

Tips for Eating Awareness

● Practice eating *slowly*! Consciously chew every bite. Consider the taste. Take a bit of chocolate or cheese and just let it dissolve on your tongue. It's better to consciously savor a small piece than to shovel in a huge amount...and face a guilty conscience.

● Eating awareness also means creating a relaxed place to dine, where you feel comfortable. Enjoy your meal. Television, newspapers, etc., can be disturbing and only distract from your body's signals. In the middle of a gripping mystery movie, would you notice that you're already full?

● Eat only when you are truly hungry and not just because it's mealtime.

● Observe yourself and learn to distinguish between real hunger and appetite. When you're hungry, you usually want something substantial. Appetite is usually associated with a craving for sweets: for example, some dessert. Who hasn't felt the urge to round off a savory meal with a taste of something sweet? So, *plan to include something sweet and enjoy it... consciously*.

● If you experience frequent cravings, become aware of which situations make you head for the cookie jar. Is it a craving? Or is it frustration, distraction, or boredom? Don't try to "eat away" your problems. Instead, try to distract yourself. Put off eating; do something fun! Go out with friends, make a hair appointment or go to a gym.

● Eat *real!* Synthetic food doesn't really satisfy, and goodness knows what the chemicals will eventually do to our systems. Eat two "real" cookies instead of a package of low-fat or no-fat cookies. In restaurants, ask for half, or kids', portions.

● Each step toward eating healthier deserves a reward. Indulge yourself, whenever you choose fresh fruit over a piece of rich, creamy cake. Give yourself a gift to motivate you to keep going.

If you've already tried all my suggestions and still can't get a grip on things, perhaps you have an eating disorder and should truly seek professional help.

Avoid Bingeing: Suggestions for In-Between Snacks

Everyone has felt it: suddenly, it's there, the feeling that you have to eat everything in the house!
You haven't eaten anything for hours, your blood sugar level is far too low and is calling for a pick-me-up. You're unable to concentrate, tired, and in a bad mood. This doesn't have to be! Planning small meals, for in-between times, saves you from being at the mercy of the eat-it-*now* attack! Make a habit of setting aside snacks that you can enjoy throughout the day, like those following. This way, your

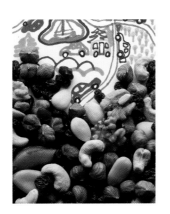

blood sugar level will remain fairly stable... and you'll feel really good!

- yogurt with fruit or cereal
- dried fruit, such as apricots
- whole grain cookies with an apple
- a cup of rice pudding
- 1 banana
- whole grain crackers with a carrot
- 1 orange or mandarin orange
- 1 glass of orange or apple juice
- baby food (no MSG, mostly pure, a perfect low-calorie snack!)

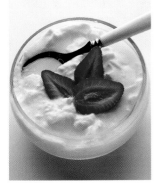

your weight you have to scale your caloric intake to your energy output. If you want to eat more, you have to increase the amount of energy you use, or in other words, become more physically active. But the number of calories burned during physical exercise has been overrated. In a half-hour of exercise you burn between 120 and 200 calories. Jogging for a half-hour only uses up 200 to 300 calories. That isn't even as much as a bar of chocolate, which has over 500 calories.

But just as with a bank account, you can adjust your energy balance. If you've spent too much, you have to save. If you went all out during the day, then all you get is a crisp salad in the evening. Indulging in a five-course meal today means being satisfied with vegetable soup or yogurt and a baked potato tomorrow.

Healthful Eating: Morning, Noon and Night

Your appointment calendar is overflowing: conference in the morning, meeting in the afternoon, workout in the evening. All too often there is no time to enjoy a meal in peace and quiet. But you should consciously take plenty of time for healthful eating. That is the foundation of healthful eating. Another point to consider: eat several small meals distributed throughout the day. Don't stuff everything into two big ones. Your daily performance curve will become much more even.

I am still amazed at the difference between American and European eating habits. Dining out in Europe is a leisurely affair that usually lasts hours. On the other hand, I often find American-style dining a bit like an assembly line. I like that the service is efficient, but I always have the feeling that they want you *out*, as fast as possible, so they can seat the next customer! So, when eating out, try to ignore meaningful stares as you sit and chew. Set a new "European" standard, and enjoy your food...*slowly*.

Start your day with breakfast. This provides you with an energy supply for the day. A good choice is cereal with fresh fruit, and milk or yogurt, or whole grain bread with a little butter or cream cheese and honey. If you can't eat anything in the morning, then you should make a habit of taking something with you to work.

In order to assure peak performance, you should eat something at lunchtime. It doesn't necessarily have to be something hot; a salad and roll are sufficient. Nowadays, all supermarkets and company dining rooms have salad bars. At work, choose foods that are good for you: vegetables, potatoes, rice, pasta, skinless poultry, fish. Skip the thick sauces and gravies.

In the evening, balance your needs by making up deficits in your eating during the day. If you ate too few fresh foods, then raw veggies or salad are called for. If you hardly had any dairy products, then baked potatoes and yogurt or whole grain bread with mozzarella and tomato are ideal. If you had too many calories, you should take that into account in the evening and, for example, just have minestrone soup and salad.

Snacks can be a source of vitamins and minerals, too. Dairy products, fruit and whole grain products are perfect. But even a cinnamon roll every now and then isn't the end of the world.

Eating Out: Guidelines for Those on the Go

Do you eat out often? Then you have the problem of choice. Should you go to the fast-food restaurant, the exclusive Italian, or the eatery next door? Keeping a few basic guidelines in mind, you can easily make the right decision. Almost all fast-food places have salad on the menu. That is the healthiest meal. But also a hamburger, which has 260 calories, is perfectly OK; just ask them to hold the mayo and french fries. After all, it contains a certain amount of iron. Pay more attention in choosing a beverage. If you decide on a can of cola (12 oz), you consume 138 calories with zero nutritional value. Instead, you should order an orange juice—its vitamin C content even promotes the absorption of iron—or a simple mineral water.

It's easy to find something healthy at the Italian restaurant. Enjoy the Mediterraneancuisine with its vegetables, olive oil, pasta and fish. You can never go wrong with pasta and tomato sauce: that makes about 200 calories. A serving of tortellini comes to about 375 calories. You can even indulge in antipastos with a clear conscience. And again, if you have a yen for soup, order some minestrone—only about 215 calories. Another tip: broiled or sautéed fish. Full meals including appetizer, main dish and dessert are often too much of a good thing. As an alternative, order two appetizers. This gives you variety and the servings are smaller. For dessert, choose fresh fruit or a light sherbet. While tiramisu, caramel custard and mousse au chocolate aren't taboo, they should remain the exception.

Asian food is an absolute pleasure and the ultimate in fitness food: lots of crisp vegetables, some rice, lean poultry or fish—and all with heavenly seasonings. Ask them to hold the MSG. It's healthier that way.

And what about the eatery next door? A serving of macaroni and cheese comes to a hefty 700 calories. More healthful choices are, again, at the salad bar. There might even be a vegetable stir-fry or salad platter. If you order meat, ask for lean broiled or sautéed dishes. Turkey and chicken are good options because the meat is very low-fat.

Drink Your Way to Health

Don't rely on your thirst. Most people have learned to suppress this sensation. Yet the body's functions depend on having enough water, because our bodies consist of almost 70% water.

Water is essential to the metabolism, for proper kidney function and for regulating body temperature through perspiration. You should take in at least 2 quarts of fluids daily. Drink at least 1½ quarts; you'll get the rest from food. For example, a cucumber

Commonly Available Menu Choices

	Calories	Carbohy-drates	Fiber	Fat	Choles-terol
Pizza with tomato, cheese, pepperoni	870	83.7	0.4	41.7	48.0
Macaroni and cheese	685	55.0	2.0	36.0	50.0
Baked beans	350	46.3	6.5	10.5	12.5
Hamburger	260	28.4	0.5	10.7	26.0
Turkey fillet, unbreaded	240	-	-	6.8	90.0
Pasta with tomato sauce	199	37.6	2.1	3.0	1.2
Baked potato	144	34.0	2.4	0.2	-

Calculations based on energy/nutritional values table by B. and H. Heseker in "Nutritional Values in Foods," Umschauverlag, Frankfurt on Main, 1993.

Calories and Nutrients in Beverages

	Calories	Carbohy-drates	Magne-sium	Vita-mins
Non-alcoholic beverages				
0.5 l apple juice spritzer	125	30.0	40.0	5.0
0.2 l vegetable juice	34	6.0	30.0	20.0
0.3 l bitter lemon	102	240	3.0	-
0.3 l cola	138	33.0	3.0	-
Alcoholic beverages				
0.5 l beer	210	12.5	45.0	-
0.5 l alcohol-free* beer	140	28.0	30.0	-
0.25 l red wine	163	0.8	20.0	5.0
0.25 l dry white wine	170	1.3	22.5	-
0.1 l champagne	72	2.8	12.0	-
50 ml sherry, dry	58	0.7	6.5	-
20 ml whisky	50	-	-	-

*Alcohol content minimal

Calculations based on energy/nutritional values table by B. and H. Heseker in "Nutritional Values in Foods," Umschauverlag, Frankfurt on Main, 1993.

Servings Guidelines

Following are some recommendations for eating well that can be used as guidelines:

● Grains, grain products, potatoes: 4 to 5 slices of whole grain bread (1½ oz.), rice or pasta (2½ to 2¾ oz.) uncooked weight), or potatoes (about 8 oz.) per day.

● Vegetables and fruit: 6½ oz. of vegetables (cooked but still crisp, to preserve the nutrients—not overcooked), 2½ oz. salad (raw) and 1 to 2 pieces of fresh fruit (about 5 to 6½ oz.) per day. Don't forget to eat legumes, too!

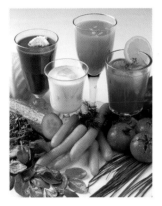

● Milk and dairy products: 4 ounces milk and 1 to 2 slices of cheese daily. If you don't like milk, choose other dairy items such as yogurt, or cottage or cream cheese.

● Fish, meat, sausage, eggs: Portions per week should be restricted to 1 to 2 servings (about 5 oz.) of ocean fish; no more than 2 to 3 servings (about 5 oz.) of meat and sausage; and no more than 3 eggs.

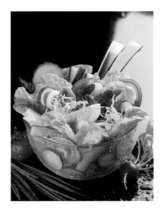

● Fats:
No more than 40g per day of cooking fat and spreads, such as 2 tablespoons of butter or margarine and 1 table spoon of oil (high-quality oil, rich in polyunsaturated fats).

Take these recommendations as guidelines. If, on some days, it doesn't work out, don't give yourself a guilty conscience. Instead, try to compensate the next day by cutting back a little—eat less in the evening and cut out the bread or rolls.

consists of 95% water, an apple is 84%, and even bread made up of 40% water.

If you perspire a lot, 1½ quarts is too little. Water lost through perspiration must be replaced in addition! You can quench your thirst without calories by drinking mineral water or herbal tea. Beverages such as vegetable and fruit juices, or buttermilk or soya can supply you with vitamins and minerals. Avoid empty calories in the form of sugar by skipping cola and other carbonated beverages. Think when you drink; after all, you have a choice.

An apple juice spritzer is a good all-around thirst quencher, after sports, too. The best mixture is three parts to one part. A spritzer not only replaces lost fluids, it also gives you potassium, which you lose through perspiration, and energy in the form of carbohydrates.

A Word about Alcohol

Remember, alcohol is an indulgence, it is not a thirst quencher! Doctor recommendations for men are to drink no more than 40mg of alcohol per day, the equivalent of about 1 liter of beer or ½ liter of wine. Women should drink even less: only half of this amount.

This is how to figure out the alcohol content of a drink: multiply the percentage on the label (percent by volume) by 0.79 (density of alcohol) and you'll get the alcohol content in grams per 100 ml. For example: If the label on a bottle of wine says "10% by volume," that means it contains 7.9g alcohol per 100 ml. That makes 79g per liter. A glass of wine (¼ l) then has just under 20g of alcohol. This is already the limit for a woman if she wants to stay fit and not overwork her liver. But there is nothing wrong with getting together and enjoying an occasional glass of wine or beer in good company.

You should also consider that, in order to digest alcohol, the body needs water. This accounts for becoming thirsty after drinking.

And if you're watching your calorie account, don't forget that a gram of alcohol has seven extra calories.

Tips for Healthful Beauty

This is how to give your body the important nutrients it needs:
● Whole grain cereal each day with fruit and milk contains carbohydrates, vitamins, and minerals as well as essential calcium.
● After every high-protein meal, eat some acidic fruit, such as oranges, lemons, kiwis, etc.

Nutritional Terms

● **Antioxidants**

By reacting with oxygen destructive agents, the so-called free radicals, can be released in foods and in the human body. Antioxidants bind these and make them harmless. Examples of natural antioxidants are: vitamins C and E. They can protect human cells from cancer. In foods, they prevent fat from becoming rancid. Artificial antioxidants (i.e. sulfites) are limited to certain foods and to certain quantities.

● **Calories (kcal)**

A unit of measure for the energy content of food. It takes one calorie to heat 1 liter of water 1 degree Centigrade. The newer unit of measure is joule. One joule is defined as the work done by a force of 1 newton applied over a distance of 1 meter in the direction of the force. 1 kcal = 4.2 kj.

● **Cholesterol**

A substance resembling fat found in foods of animal origin such as egg yolk, butter, meat, organ meats and sausage. If you consume too much of it, your level of blood cholesterol rises. The consequences are arteriosclerosis and increased risk of heart attack.

The following substances reduce the level of blood cholesterol: polyunsaturated fats (in plant oils such as safflower, sunflower, corn and soy), and fiber (i.e. soluble fiber in oat germ) or pectin in apples. Physical exercise also has a positive effect on blood fat values.

Blood cholesterol levels for adults are defined as:

Desirable	<200 mg/dl
Borderline-high	200-239 mg/dl
High	240 mg/dl and above

● **Distilled Water**

Distilled water has had all the minerals removed from it! Because of this, it robs the body of vital minerals as it is eliminated.

Possible consequences: cardiovascular disorders, headache, muscle cramps. Instead: drink mineral water or tap water.

● **Enzymes**

These biocatalysts in our bodies initiate the metabolism and digestion. Enzymes consist of protein and often work only in combination with vitamins, minerals and trace elements. Our food also contains plenty of enzymes exotic fruits such as pineapple or papaya. Enzyme derivatives made from them are often touted as miracle diets. But unfortunately, the miracle of pounds that disappear by themselves never happens. To really get rid of fat deposits there is only one way: eat right, drink right and exercise!

● **Glycogen**

The reservoir of carbohydrates in the body, stored in the liver and muscles.

● **HDL and LDL**

HDL and LDL are two types of lipoproteins. They are manufactured by the body to tranport fat and cholesterol through the blood. LDLs, or low-density lipoproteins, contain the greatest amounts of cholesterol and may be the culprit for depositing cholesterol on the artery walls. This is why LDLs are often referred to as the "bad" cholesterol. LDL cholesterol levels 160 mg/dl and above are classified as high risk. LDL levels can also be lowered by exercise, weight loss and proper nutrition.

HDL's, or high-density lipoproteins, contain more protein than cholesterol. They help remove cholesterol from the cells in the arteries and transport it back to the liver for elimination from the body. That's why they're often called the "good" cholesterol. Levels of HDL cholesterol below 35 mg/dl are classified as high risk.

The total cholesterol : HDL *ratio* is a more precise indicator of risk than the total cholesterol. The higher the ratio, the greater the risk of coronary heart disease. For example:

Total cholesterol = 140mg/dl

HDL = 30 mg/dl

Ratio = 240/30 = 8.0 (a high-risk ratio)

Ideal ratio for men: <4.0

Ideal ratio for women: <3.5

● Hydrogenation (trans fatty acids)

This is a process where hydrogen atoms are added to monounsaturated and polyunsaturated oils. Oils are hydrogenated for two reasons, increased shelf life and improved texture. Hydrogenated fats affect the body in much the same way as saturated fats. They are responsible for increasing the levels of LDL cholesterol. Some studies have shown that trans fatty acids posed a greater risk to the heart than saturated fats found in meats and dairy food. Conversely, some studies have shown that trans fats result in lower blood cholesterol levels than saturated fats. So research goes on. I suggest prudence and eating naturally as the best solution!

● Hypoglycemia (low blood sugar)

Hypoglycemia during sports. The cause: the liver's glycogen reserve is empty so blood sugar cannot be maintained at a constant level. Possible consequences are sudden cravings, dizziness, weakness and fatigue.

Here is how to prevent hypoglycemia: Before sports activities, eat something high in carbohydrates (pasta, potatoes, bread). Keep carbohydrate-rich sports snacks, such as bananas, dried fruit or granola bars, handy.

● Lactate

Lactic acid is a waste product of anaerobic energy production and is produced in the muscles during high intensity, short bouts of exercise like sprinting. If lactic acid is produced faster than it can be eliminated, muscle fatigue results.

● Meat

Though it contains high-quality protein and iron, too much meat is unhealthy. You can survive entirely without meat if your meal plan provides for sufficient legumes, whole grain products, sprouts and potatoes.

● Osteoporosis

A loss of bone density occurring mainly in women after menopause as a result of estrogen deficiency. Prevention can begin early: make sure you consume enough calcium. It is recommended that a menopausal woman take 1,500 mg daily. Milk and cheese are good sources, but if you don't like or can't tolerate them, choose vegetables like broccoli, turnips and plenty of green leafy salads. Engage in weight bearing exercises like walking and begin a strength training program. Women should have bone density checks by age forty and then regularly at least every two years.

● Overweight

Overweight is defined as being 10% over the average weight according to standard height/weight charts. However, up to date research tells us that our percentage of body fat is farm more important in determining good health and good body composition. You can even be considered thin and still be "overfat." Muscles weight more than fat, so if you do a lot of strength training, you might be very lean with good to excellent body fat levels, but weight more than someone your height who has poor or high body fat levels.

● Underweight

Is defined as being 10% below the average weight according to the standard height/weight charts. However, it is far more important to know your percentage of body fat. For a woman, levels below 15% could be far too low to maintain good health.

Body fat norms for adults are given as:

	Male	Female
Very lean	<8%	<15%
Healthy	8–12	18–22
Obese	>20%	>30%

VIII. Music to Train By

Music is an incredible motivational tool. I *need* music to exercise—it never ceases to give me energy when I have none.

Music not only determines the tempo of the movements we make, it creates an atmosphere and has a stimulating and encouraging effect on us.

Music uplifts us and makes us work harder. It makes exercising a pleasure instead of a drudge. If you're listening to your favorite cassette or CD, you can set little goals for yourself. For example, 3 songs for the warm-up, or stay on the treadmill for half the CD or cassette.

Many clients have asked me to explain simply how workout music is constructed, i.e., how rhythms are used in aerobic training. In aerobics, we work in beats of 8 to a phrase. I like to think of this as a sentence. We start out on the 1 and end on the 8. The speed or tempo of the music is measured in beats per minute (bpm). If you listen well and practice counting, you will be able to identify the first beat of the phrase. Working in time with the music is even more motivating.

Choosing Your Own Movin' Music

Choice of music is a very personal matter. Nowadays, you can even purchase tailor-made aerobic cassettes or CDs with top 40 hits or oldies, or hip-hop cassettes for step, workout, low or mixed impact training, etc. Music for warm-ups should not be too fast (a step cassette is a good choice).

The question now is, what kind of training is for you? If it's cardiovascular, you'll want peppy, inspiring music, maybe even a little aggressive, to get the fire going. The beat should be strong and accented. The tempo should be fast enough to encourage a similar heart rate, but it must also accommodate your movements. If it makes you run or jump too slowly, you'll tire more easily and will feel that you are being weighed down. If it's too fast, you won't be able to keep up the pace and your technique will be the first to go.

After your cardiovascular training, the bpm should gradually be decreased until your heart rate has fallen at least 30 beats (never, *ever*, stop abruptly!). When working out for muscle strength and endurance, make sure the music inspires strength and power, but that it is slow enough to allow for full range of motion and clean technique. For stretching purposes, slow, fluid music that allows for complete relaxation is a perfect choice. Because your stretches are static and should be held for longer intervals, music without a recognizable beat is the best bet!

With music everything is easier. Music motivates and makes each workout a fun experience. With the right music, time seems to fly by; this means you'll stick with your cardio-endurance or muscle workout longer. Set a goal for yourself when training for cardio-endurance: first just one song, then keep going for two, then three. Do this regularly over weeks, each week adding one more song to your training session! With discipline and the right music, you'll reach your goals sooner than you thought you could.

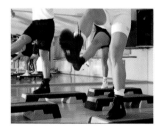

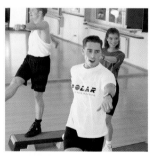

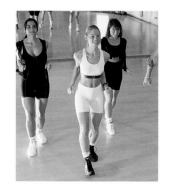

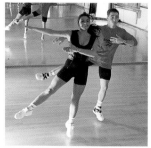

Jennifer's Favorites

Here are a few examples of music I like and find appropriate for different workouts:

● **For muscle strength and endurance and step training, music with a bpm tempo of 118–126, such as:**
"Because of Love" – Janet Jackson
"Pressure" – Michael and Janet Jackson
"Dream Lover" – Mariah Carey
"Eye of the Tiger" – Survivor

● **For low-impact, slide, or walking (on a treadmill); music with a bpm of 120–145, such as:**
"It's Raining Men" – Weather Girls
"Don't Cry for Me Argentina" – Madonna
"Nutbush City Limits" – Tina Turner

●**For mixed or high-impact training or running (on a treadmill); music with a bpm of 145–165, such as:**
"Power of Love" – Sylvester
"Take Me To Heaven" – Sylvester
"Looking for a Hero" – Bonnie Tyler

Almost all songs from Madonna are great for muscle or low-impact training. Funk and soul music complement muscle workouts as well. Hard rock fans can use it for inspiring high-impact or running sessions. The so-called "techno" sound releases just the right endorphins for some people—it can be especially motivating for stationary cycling. Some love classical pop, or find the cancan or other energetic folk dances inspiring for cardio-vascular endurance workouts. Classical, esoteric and meditational music are wonderful for relaxing and stretching. The composer Kitaro is one of my own favorites.

Talking Volumes

Music is emotion for me. Without it, my life would not be what it is. Most of us feel this way. A sad song will evoke a memory of a lost love or a beautiful moment. A top 40 hit from 1977 will make us remember an unforgettable summer holiday.

Unfortunately, music can also be annoying, disturbing, or even damaging. If you play your CD too loud, a neighbor might be less than enthusiastic, and if you work out or take aerobic classes where the music reaches mega decibels, you might not find it very inspiring—or *you* might, but your eardrums won't thank you. Listening to music through earphones with the volume turned all the way up is very damaging to your ears—so if you want to enjoy music for years to come, watch the volume!

Well, now you know all you need to, so let's get started on a new chapter in your life. Enjoy getting healthier, stronger and more active every day. Keep it up and success will be yours.

Glossary

Abduction   away from the median of the body or limb

Adduction   toward the median of the body or limb

Aerobic   (oxidative) in the presence of oxygen

Agonist   the prime mover, the muscle primarily responsible for producing the movement

Alignment   the line of the body in certaom positions or movements

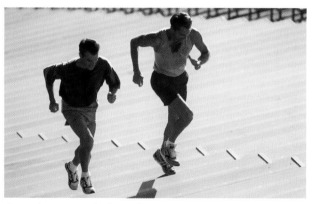

A good way to train for endurance.

Anaerobic   (anoxidative) not in the presence of oxygen

Antagonist   the muscle which opposes the prime mover

Atrophy   degeneration, as of muscle tissue

Ball   portion of foot behind the toes; a stance with the weight on the balls of the feet, with heels lifted

Biomechanics   literally, "life movements": a science of human movement (kinesiology) particularly the in-depth study of the mechanical aspects

Bodysculpting   also "bodyshaping," "bodystyling"—all names for muscle strength group fitness classes

Burnout   a phenomenon of over-training; too much physical or psychological stress can cause this drastic drop in performance (*see* Overtraining)

Cellulite   Subcutaneous fat cells that give the skin an orange peel appearance. Usually on thighs, upper arms, stomach.

Contraction   tensing and shortening of a muscle; the muscle "shrinks together"

Contraindicated   not a good idea! In group fitness, the expression "contraindicated exercise" means one that is not recommended, usually because it is considered a high risk. For example: windmills; plow; forward, fully flexed kneebends without support; extended leg sit-ups into sitting position; jackknife; hurdler's stretch; etc.

Crunch   an abdominal exercise where the emphasis is on the abdominal muscles squeezing or "crunching" together

Curl   an abdominal exercise; the upper body leaves the floor

Double-duty   one exercise simultaneously training two muscle groups

Dynamic   from the Greek word for "powerful"; a form of muscle contraction in which the muscle shortens

Enzymes   proteins, occurring in living organisms, which accelerate chemical reactions

Expiration   exhalation

Fat burner   an aerobic class taught in steady state to promote the burn-off of body fat.

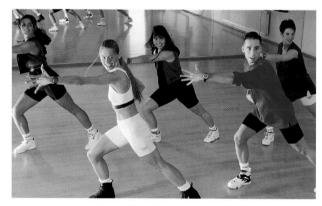

Aerobics can be almost like dancing.

Footwrap   a method of winding tubing around the foot for the purposes of training

Hamstrings   the muscle groups running down the back of the legs that cause them to flex

Heart rate   heartbeats per minute (*see* Target heart rate)

High impact impacted movements, where both feet leave the ground, such as while running, jumping, leaping, hopping

Hip-hop a variation of aerobics especially appropriate for the younger set. The term comes from the music scene

Hyperextension/Hyperflexion overstretching/overextending, a joint being moved past its normal extension

Hyperlordosis extreme curvature of the spine in the lumbar region

Hypertrophy extreme increase in tissue size, for example thickening of the muscle

Impact movements distinguished according to degree of biomechanical stress (see High impact and Low impact)

Impingement refers to the impingement syndrome or "pinching" of the shoulder tissues

Inspiration inhalation

Isometric (static) although tension is created, there is no movement at the joint

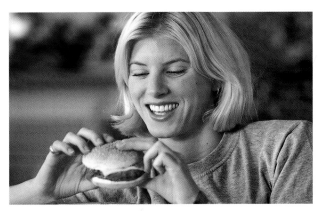

Perfectly OK: the occasional hamburger.

Isotonic (dynamic) there is joint movement and tension is generated. There are two types of isotonic contractions: *concentric*—in which the muscle shortens; and *eccentric*—in which the muscle lengthens

Kyphosis curvature of the spine in the thoracic region

Lactate a salt in milk acid that is detectable in the blood

Lateral sideways

Lordosis curvature of the spine in the lumbar and cervical regions

Low impact movements in which at least one foot always remains on the floor; such as in the process of marching. Because the impact, or force at landing, is much lower than high-impact training, there is less risk of certain injuries.

Luxation dislocation of a joint

Medial medial, central

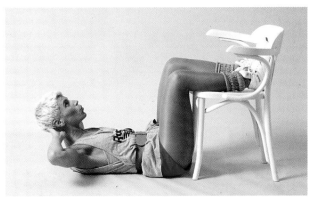

For your good looks: abdominal exercises.

Mixed-impact both high- and low-impact movements

Muscle tone the natural tension a muscle has at rest

Overload the use of more resistance or repetitions. By doing overloading, we challenge the muscle to work harder than it is used to, so it will adapt. The principle is called progressive training.

Over-training the human body cannot be trained infinitely; it needs resting phases in order to regenerate itself and be ready to perform again. A form of "burnout," symptoms of over-training include: restlessness, irritability, lack of concentration, decreased physical performance and cardiovascular disorders.

Personal trainer someone knowledgeable who is able to direct and instruct a client in a schedule of individualized workouts with a goal of physical fitness

Placement distribution of body weight in certain positions or movements

Pull-up special muscle exercise for the biceps

Push-up traditional exercise for chest and triceps

Reverse crunch an abdominal exercise; the lower abdominal section squeezes or crunches towards the upper section

Reverse curl an abdominal exercise; the lower body leaves the floor

Rotation turning or twisting

Scoliosis sideways curvature of the spine

Sequence the order of movements within an exercise

Set an established number of repetitions of a strength exercise

Slide an athletic form of training done by gliding on a special mat; the sideways motions resemble that of speed skating

Spinning a trademark name for cardiovascular training on indoor stationary cycles to music

Static an exercise without any dynamic movement

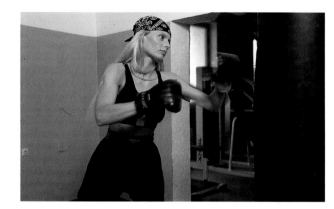

Reach out!—Go for it!

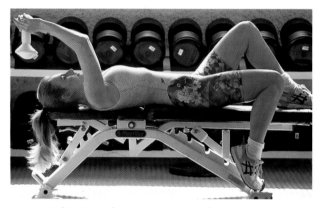

Free weights strengthen your arm muscles.

Steady state the training state in which equilibrium between energy output and supply has been achieved

Step form of aerobics using steps (platforms); stepping up and down trains the lower body; the accompanying vigorous arm movements train the upper body

Target heart rate a recommended value of 60–75% of the maximum attainable heart rate; this is the pulse range during endurance training

Tubing elastic band with handles, for use in exercising

Warm-up a series of movements designed to prepare the body for upcoming training; it should last 6–10 minutes at least

Workout another term for training

Acknowledgments

First and foremost, I thank my dear friend and colleague, Ute Haas. This book could not have happened without you.

Thanks to Lyne Bils for the great translation—you were a life saver.

To Claire Bazinet, thank you for your patience and perseverance. You really know how to make my words work!

How could I have achieved what I did without your belief in me?— My crusaders at Reebok Germany, Astrid Foerster, who "discovered" me and my "baby," Barbara Ebersberger, who is now my boss!

Bernhard Pichler, you gave me the freedom to develop all my crazy ideas.

To all my dear colleagues at Leo's Sports Club who support my philosophy and help me live my ideals.

Thanks to Suedwest Verlag, and especially Stefanie, who spent so many hours working on the original text.

To Polar Germany, who has the vision to "Find the Balance."

To Icon Health and Fitness, Germany, who know that "personal training" is the future fitness.

And how could I forget my clients and my students, who challenge me and keep me growing

To my Uncle Bob, who has always been there to help when others have not.

And my brother, Sam, who predicted a future in fitness for me, before "fitness" existed.

To my two daughters, for showing me what life is all about.

And last but not least, to my wonderful husband, Stephen, who has gone through thick and thin with me. I am what I am because of the love he has given me.